12.95

D0931053

⋯§DRUG〰

ANTIQUES

A Photographic Look at Old and Unusual Drug Artifacts and Rarities

With Current Values and an Introduction

⋯§JED POWER〰

CAPE ANN ANTIQUES
Peabody, MA 01960

Copyright © 1986 by James H. Power

All rights reserved. No part of this book may be reproduced or
transmitted in any form or by any means, electronic or mechanical,
including photocopying, recording or by any information storage or
retrieval system—except by a reviewer who may quote brief passages
in a review to be printed in a magazine or newspaper—without
permission in writing from the publisher. For information contact
Cape Ann Antiques, P. O. Box 3502, Peabody, MA 01960.

First Printing 1986

Library of Congress Catalog Card Number: 86-71264

ISBN 0-9616832-0-1

The current values in this book should be used only as a guide. They
are not intended to set prices. Prices vary greatly and are affected by
condition and demand. The author and publisher assume no
responsibility for any losses that might be incurred as a result of using
this book.

Printed in the United States of America.

For Candy, Courtney, Jackie and Tim

❧ CONTENTS ☙

❦INTRODUCTION❧

This book is not intended as an indepth look at drug antiques or the drug collectibles field. It is intended only to show those not familiar with this field the wide range of items which are collected and also to give a very general idea of their values. Also, some other very basic and helpful topics about this collecting area are discussed.

Although this book is aimed at the uninitiated, those with more expertise in this field will also find it enjoyable, if for no other reason than that this book is the first written concerning the drug antiques and collectibles field. More advanced collectors will also enjoy the chance to look at photographs of many different drug artifacts which otherwise they may never have had the opportunity to see. Also, this book will be helpful as a reference guide.

All price values in this book are based upon items in very good condition, unless otherwise stated.

WHAT ARE DRUG ANTIQUES?

Drug antiques and collectibles are comprised of almost anything to do with psychoactive drugs such as marijuana, cocaine, coca, opiates and psychedelics.

INTRODUCTION

The items collected include bottles, books, tins, magazines, posters, documents and advertising, to name only a few. They range in size from 3″ × 5″ Vin Mariani Coca Wine postcards to a life-size wax oriental opium smoker (which I was once offered the chance to purchase).

Drug antiques come from all eras, although the majority do come from three time periods.

The first is the 1880–1914 period when America had its great drug-use explosion. Thousands of concoctions containing opiates, cocaine and cannabis were churned out during this time span. Left behind, for future collectors, were countless empty drug bottles and tins. As problems with these drugs began to arise so did the literature on this controversial subject increase, until the popular press of the day was filled with drug-related stories and editorials. Countless books on the subject were also published. This debate culminated with passage of the 1914 Harrison Narcotics Act which brought an end to the flood of narcotic-containing products on the over-the-counter market. Interest in the topic died down, and the number of writings on drug use declined dramatically.

The second phase encompassed the years 1930–1953. Though not as significant as the first stage, these years nonetheless left behind countless drug collectibles mostly of the literary kind. The 1930's decade saw a heated public discussion over marijuana, which escalated into the passage of the Marijuana Tax Act of 1937. Again, the press churned out myriad articles on the matter. The 1940's and early 1950's brought a blizzard of anti-drug articles and books from publishers. It was a time of highly sensationalized reporting on the drug topic.

The third stage is the second great drug explosion which is occurring now. Beginning in the early 1960's, this era closely resembles the 1880-1914 years (though we will not get into that here). Because of the illegality of drugs, this period is producing a mountain of literature and ephemera and very little in the way of bottles, tins, etc. In the future, much of the paraphernalia manufactured during this time such as rolling machines, coke spoons, etc., may have value, but right now they are too common and rarely collected— though this will change as time passes.

The desirability of collectibles from these times pretty much co-incide with their age. The turn of the century antiques, being the most valuable, followed by the 1930–1953 pieces, with the current group being least costly. This is not a hard and fast rule though. There are some exceptions. Several one hundred-year-old objects are very common and not highly priced; while on the other hand there are some very scarce and valuable collectibles to be found from the 1960's.

WHO COLLECTS DRUG ANTIQUES?

A large cross section of people are involved in the drug collectibles field. Doctors, lawyers, pharmacists, researchers, and people from almost all other walks of life are enthusiastic collectors. Also people involved on all sides of the controversial drug issues of the day are avid collectors.

Some of the most extensive collections are owned, and expanded regularly, by the world's largest drug companies. Many of these huge conglomerates trace their origins back to founders who amassed great fortunes by manufacturing and distributing these drugs before the turn of the century.

Many collectors came of age during the 1960's and had their interest in psychoactive drugs stimulated by the mores of that decade. Out of curiosity, they delved into the history of these drugs. Through their research and coinciding personal experiences of themselves and those around them, more than a few came to the realization of the possible dangers of some of these substances. Though they may have altered their personal relationship with these drugs, many never lost their interest in them and in their fascinating history.

INTRODUCTION

WHY COLLECT DRUG ANTIQUES?

Drug antiques are collected for many different reasons—the foremost being personal enjoyment. As in any collectible field, the people involved in collecting drug antiques derive satisfaction from possessing something old and historically significant. They find it fulfilling to seek out new and desirable items for their collections. There is as much enjoyment in the hunt for new items as in their actual ownership.

Also because drugs are such a topical subject today, the collector has a unique bird's eye view on the overall history that has led to one of the most controversial social questions of our day.

Another reason for collecting is, of course, the investment potential. Although the collectibles field generally can be a volatile market with many ups and downs, there is one period in any collectible area when all prices rise dramatically. This is in the beginning stage of a new collectible field. During this phase, early collectors can acquire quality items at relatively inexpensive prices. As the field grows and receives wider media attention, more people will be attracted to collecting in it. Collector competition will gradually grow fierce, forcing prices up spectacularly. Investors can only take advantage of a situation of this type if they enter a relatively new field still in its infancy. This is the stage I believe the drug antiques and collectibles field is now in. The number of people involved is increasing, and the press is showing interest including some major national outlets such as "Life," "Playboy," and others. Already I have seen items being sold for two and three times what they were selling for less than a year ago. I would advise any would-be investor to stick with quality items in at least very good or near mint condition. These better grades have always shown the greatest appreciation potential.

Also there are no guarantees in any collectible field, so try to accumulate things which you will enjoy having even if the financial aspects are not as rewarding as you feel they will be. That way no matter what happens, you will not be a loser.

INTRODUCTION

WHERE TO FIND DRUG ANTIQUES

There are many avenues to take in your search for drug antiques and collectibles. Some can be quite productive, while others like flea markets, are not really worth the large amounts of time invested.

The following are a few of the more fertile areas in which to conduct your search.

Show Dealers

Today there are all types of shows held in all parts of the country. There are bottle shows, paper collectible shows, and general collectible shows, among others. These shows, which sometimes have hundreds of dealers selling their goods, are often excellent places to seek out drug antiques and collectibles.

The trick in being successful in your search at these shows, is being able to wade quickly through the mountains of material that you are not interested in. Do not get bogged down at a table or in a group of items which are unlikely to have any drug-related material. Pick the most promising looking stalls to search through first. You can always hit the others on your return. Although the time and effort expended at a show can be great, it is almost always rewarded with at least a few interesting finds.

Show dates can be found in most general antique and collectible publications and in the more specialized periodicals concerning their own fields. A few helpful publications are listed at the end of this chapter.

Collector Publications

Another area to consider in your quest are the various publications devoted to antiques and collectibles.

Some, such as the ANTIQUE TRADER WEEKLY, are quite general, covering every type of collectible imaginable. Most of these type of periodicals have extensive classified advertising sections. A

INTRODUCTION

careful search of sections relevant such as books, bottles, magazines, etc., will often turn up sellers with interesting items for sale.

Even more helpful are the specialized collectible magazines put out concerning specific fields. There are ones involved in bottles, books, magazines, paper, posters and almost anything else you can imagine.

Again, some of these periodicals are listed at the end of this chapter.

Mail-Order Dealers

Although at this time there is only one mail-order dealer who specializes in drug antiques and collectibles (name and address at the end of this chapter), there are others who have more than the average amount of drug antiques among their general stock.

Your best bet on finding dealers who carry some drug collectibles among their wares is to check ads in the antique publications and also to check through catalogs on display at shows you attend. Also, other collectors may be able to point you in the right direction. Get yourself on the mailing list of any dealers who seem to carry some drug-related material.

When purchasing from mail-order dealers, always trade with ones who are reliable and who offer a one-hundred percent money-back guarantee. This is especially important concerning mail order, where purchases are mostly made sight unseen.

Other Collectors

Often times coming in contact with other collectors will lead to new additions for your collection.

You may find that you have something another collector wants and that a trade can be worked out for a desirable piece from his/her collection.

Other times collectors will be interested in selling varying portions of their collections, either because of duplicate items, financial reasons, or for one of many other causes.

Knowing other collectors in the drug antiques area will be extremely beneficial not only for the aforementioned, but also as a way to keep abreast of important information and trends in this collectible field.

Self-Advertising

Self-advertising is another excellent way to acquire drug antiques.

Most of the general and speciality collectible magazines have a reasonably priced classified section. Often a small, well written want ad in one of these publications will generate some interesting offers.

Remember, be specific in your description of your wants. A reference to drug antiques only will often bring letters offering more general medical, dental and pharmaceutical antiques. Mention the drugs you are interested in; i.e., marijuana, cocaine, etc.

Also, be sure to place your ad in the right type of publication. If you are interested in bottles, you will do the best advertising, obviously, in a bottle magazine rather than in a book collectors' publication or a general collectibles periodical.

Remember, acquiring antiques in this way will enable you to get them for a more reasonable price. You have overhead to consider (advertising cost, etc.) and also you are buying, for the most part, directly from the source and not dealers.

Again, a list of possible publications for self-advertising follows.

The following is a list of companies and publications which are useful, to one degree or another, in locating drug antiques and collectibles:

Cape Ann Antiques
P. O. Box 3502
Peabody, MA 01960

This is the first and, as of this writing, the only business specializing exclusively in drug antiques and collectibles. They have a catalog available for $2.00.

INTRODUCTION

The Antique Trader Weekly
P. O. Box 1050
Dubuque, Iowa 52001

A general antiques publication, in newspaper format, with a very large circulation. They have an extensive and reasonably-priced classified section which carries all types of antiques.

The Antique Bottle Collector
Box 187
East Greenville, PA 18041

A bottle collector publication which also has a good classified section.

The Paper and Advertising Collector
P. O. Box 500
Mount Joy, PA 17552

A publication, with a large classified section, devoted to all kinds of paper collectibles.

American Book Collector
P. O. Box 867
Ossining, NY 10562

A book collectors' magazine with a classified section.

CONDITION GRADING OF DRUG ANTIQUES

One of the most important aspects of any antique or collectible is its physical condition. This can have a major effect on an item's worth and desirability.

Drug antiques, having originated from many collectible fields

INTRODUCTION

such as bottles, books, and ephemera, have incorporated something from the grading systems of all of these fields into their own grading structure.

The following are the most common gradings, in use today, of drug antiques and collectibles:

Poor: Item has major damage

Fair: Heavy wear and/or moderate damage

Good: Moderate to heavy wear and/or use markings

Very Good: Minor to moderate wear and/or use markings

Near Mint: Very slight wear and/or use markings

Mint: Like new. No visible wear or use markings.

Occasionally, especially in mail order, you will run across some pieces which have been given a dual rating; i.e., a book jacket could have heavy damage and be rated poor, while the book itself could have very slight wear and be classified in near mint condition. Or a bottle could be in very good or near mint condition, while the bottle label could be heavily worn or obscured and be graded fair or poor.

Also, you may see some items which are given a rating with a reservation; i.e., "label has small corner piece missing with no text loss, otherwise bottle in near mint condition."

All of these practices are acceptable if their outcome is a better understanding by all concerned of a collectible's true condition.

Most collectors will see very few mint pieces available and, hopefully, even fewer items in poor or fair condition.

It is advisable, when adding to your collection, to stick with collectibles in at least good condition and, better still, to acquire objects in very good or near mint condition only.

INTRODUCTION

The only time a collector should consider purchasing an antique in poor or fair condition is when the collectible is unique or extremely rare or when higher grades of a particular piece are no longer available.

An understanding of these condition categories will help immeasurably in making wise purchases of drug antiques and will be invaluable in mail order situations where a collectible is often purchased sight unseen.

CONCENTRATING YOUR COLLECTION

Many collectors tend to limit their collecting to one specific area. This is done for a couple of different reasons. Some collectors find that there are too many items available and that if they bought everything they liked, budget permitting, they would have little more than a hodge podge of minimally-related collectibles. Other collectors find that their interests are focused on one distinct subject or type of collectible.

Collectors have concentrated their collections in many different directions. There are collections comprised of specific kinds of collectibles. Whole collections of nothing but drug-related books exist. Others enjoy collecting bottles, magazines, paper or any other of a number of different types of antiques.

Many collections contain all types of collectibles but zero in on one category of drug, such as marijuana, cocaine or opiates.

Some collectors have combined both by collecting only marijuana-related books for example.

Collections are often built around one or more famous people. Timothy Leary, for one, is the center of several collections.

Often collections are built around a timeframe—such as pieces from the 1960's. Or collections containing pre-1914 Harrison Act collectibles only.

Others just like to acquire high-quality items only, no matter what they may be.

Whatever a collection revolves around, focusing in one area will give a collection a sense of direction and cohesiveness.

AVOIDING FAKES!

One of the good points of the drug antique field being in its early stages is that it has yet to attract any significant amount of counterfeiters. Because counterfeiters like to palm off their goods easily and quickly, for big bucks, these con men gravitate to the antique fields which have already peaked, and are loaded with literally thousands of possible avenues to dispose of their goods and millions of unwary buyers ready to throw their money away.

Unfortunately, as the drug antiques field grows, undoubtedly so will the number of fakes to be found gradually increase.

Common sense is the greatest protection you have against being stuck with a fraudulent antique or collectible.

It is a good idea to be wary of any item that seems to be too good to be true, especially coming from a supposedly knowledgeable source. Check it out thoroughly, or find someone who can verify its authenticity for you. Maybe you have stumbled across an underpriced goodie—but better safe than sorry.

Mint and near mint items should always be given a very careful going over. Although some genuine mint items do exist, if it looks like it is brand new, maybe it is! Again, check it thoroughly yourself or have it checked out.

Enscribed books, in the drug antiques field, will probably see their share of fakes. Ask the seller where he got the book. Trace it back. Does it make any sense with what you know of the activities of the signer? You would be surprised how many books have been enscribed and dated by an author who was dead or incapacitated at that time.

Bottles of new vintage may have old labels or xerox copies of old labels pasted on them. Notice if the bottle appears to be of a more recent making than the label indicates it should.

INTRODUCTION

Some areas will most likely have very little counterfeiting activity, such as inexpensive embossed bottles, magazines and items that are not profitable or practical for the counterfeiter to duplicate.

The best way of protecting yourself is by always dealing with reputable dealers. Although a dealer, too, can sometimes be fooled, a reputable one will always make amends for an item of this type that he has sold. This is especially important in dealing with mail-order distributors, considering that you will be buying a collectible without having seen it first.

If you follow these suggestions and do not leave your common sense at home when shopping for drug antiques, you will never be a counterfeiter's victim.

BOOKS

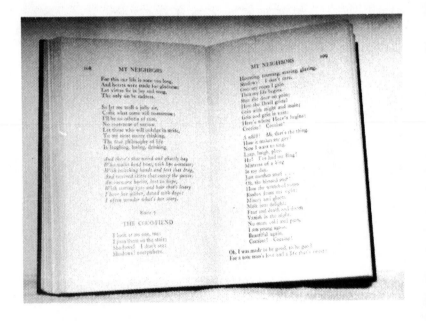

Ballads of a Bohemian

by Robert Service Hard. Contains six-page poem: *The Coco-Fiend.* (*I am young again, beautiful again. Cocaine! Cocaine!*) Also seven-page poem: *The Absinthe Drinker.* 1st edition, 1921. Hardcover, 220 pages. $50.00

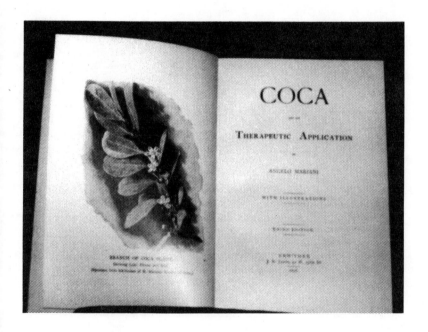

Coca and Its Therapeutic Application
by Angelo Mariani. 3rd edition, 1896. 77 pages with illustrations. $60.00

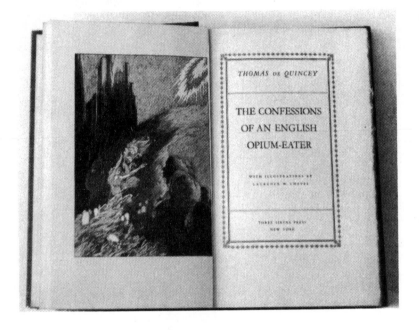

Confessions of an English Opium Eater
by Thomas DeQuincy. 1932, Three Sirens Press edition. 228
pages with illustrations by Laurence Chaves. Hardcover. $35.00

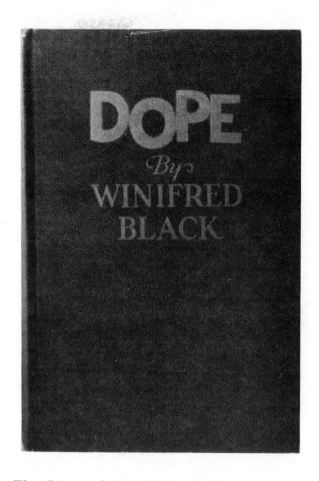

Dope, The Story of the Living Dead
by Winifred Black. 1st edition, 1928. Hardcover, 104 pages.
$45.00

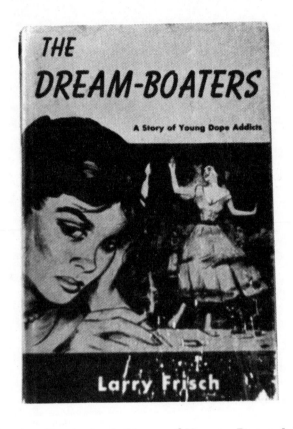

The Dream-Boaters, A Story of Young Dope Addicts
by Larry Frisch. 1st edition, 1953. Hardcover with dustjacket.
122 pages. $45.00

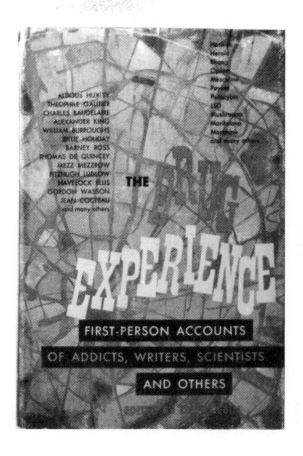

The Drug Experience—First-Person Accounts of Addicts, Writers, Scientists and Others
by David Elbin. 1st edition, 1961. Hardcover with dustjacket. 384 pages. $25.00

BOOKS

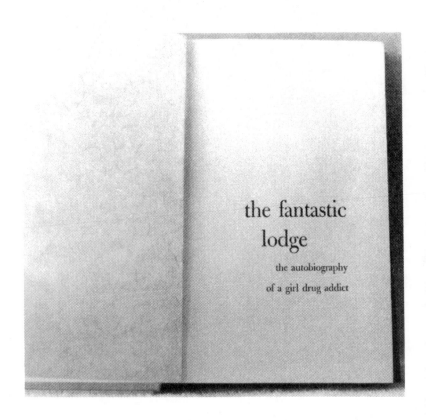

The Fantastic Lodge—Autobiography of a Girl Drug Addict
by Helen Hughes. 1st printing, 1961. Hardcover, 267 pages.
$35.00

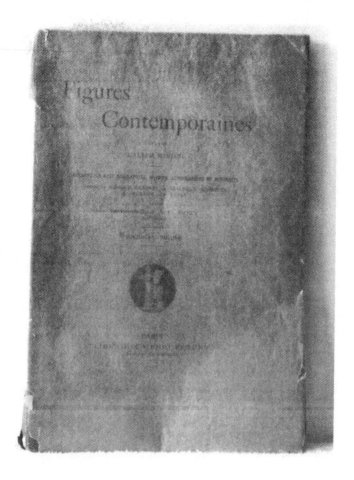

Figures Contemporaines
Volume 5, 1900. Papercover. Contains illustrations of and testimonials by famous people of the day praising Vin Mariani Coca Wine. $60.00

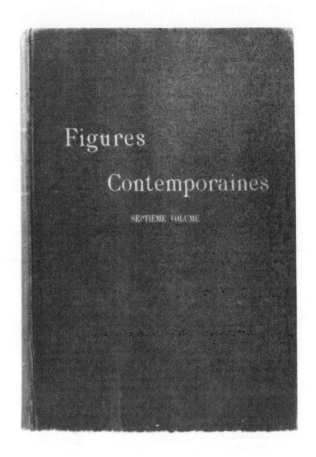

Figures Contemporaines
Volume 7, 1902. Hardcover. Contains illustrations of and
testimonials by famous people of the day praising Vin Mariani
Coca Wine. $80.00

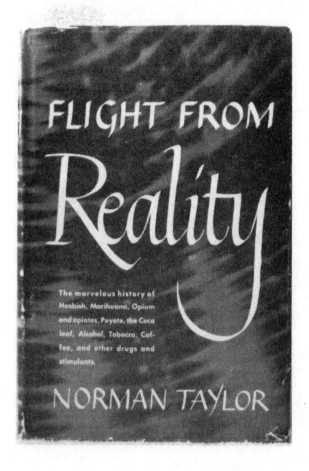

Flight From Reality—The Marvelous History of Hashish, Marijuana, Opium, Coca Leaf . . ., etc. by Norman Taylor. 1st edition, 1949. Hardcover with dustjacket. 237 pages. $45.00

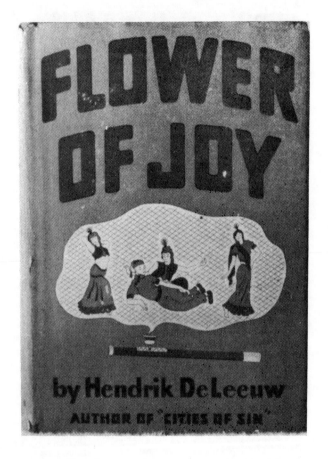

Flower of Joy
by Hendrick DeLeeuw. 1st edition, 1939. Hardcover with
dustjacket. 241 pages. $30.00

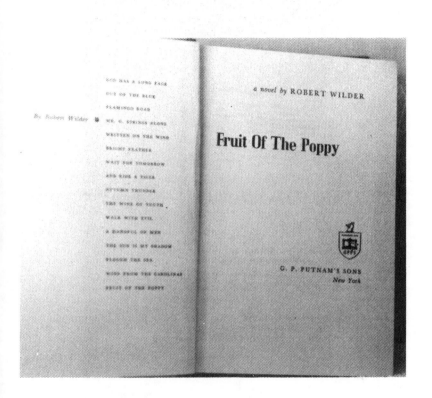

Fruit of the Poppy
by Robert Wilder. 1st edition, 1965. Hardcover, 252 pages.
$25.00

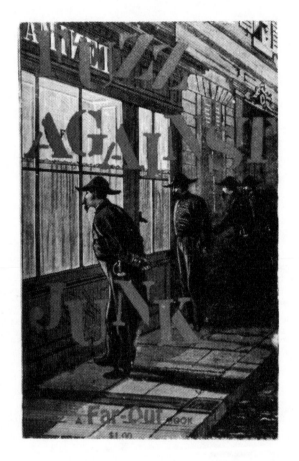

Fuzz Against Junk—the Saga of the Narcotics Brigade
by Akbar del Piombo. 1st American edition, 1961. 92 pages with illustrations. Papercover. $25.00

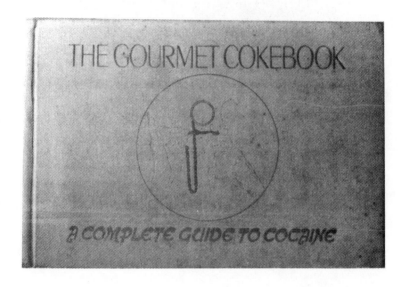

The Gourmet Cokebook—A Complete Guide to Cocaine
2nd edition, 1972. Hardcover, 97 pages. White Mountain Press. $35.00

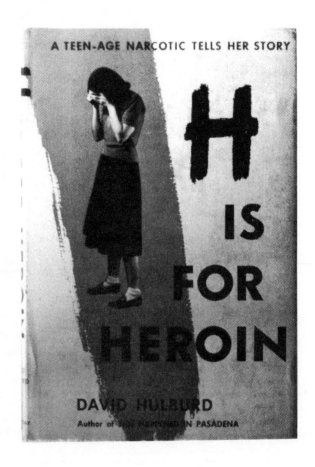

H is for Heroin—A Teenage Narcotic Tells Her Story
by David Hulburd. 1st edition, 1952. Hardcover with dustjacket.
122 pages. $25.00

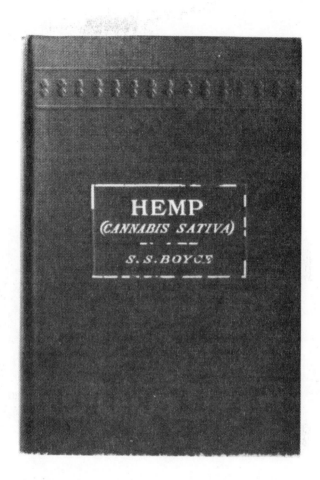

Hemp (Cannabis Sativa)—A Practical Treatise on the
Culture of Hemp Seed and Fiber With a Sketch of
History and Nature of Hemp Plant
by S.S. Boyce. Copyright 1900, 1912 edition. Hardcover. 112
pages with photos and illustrations. $45.00

BOOKS

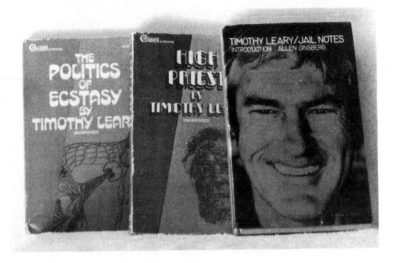

Three books by Timothy Leary. Left to right:
1. *The Politics of Ecstasy*, Papercover, 1968. $30.00;
2. *High Priest*, 1st print, 1968. Papercover. $25.00;
3. *Jail Notes*, 1st print, 1970. Hardcover with dustjacket. $30.00

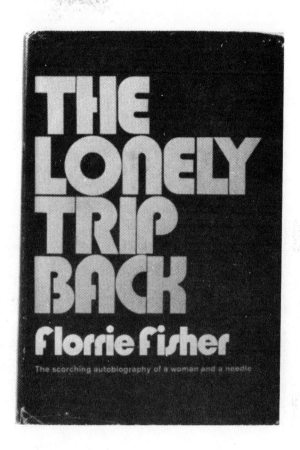

The Lonely Trip Back
by Florrie Fisher. 1st edition, 1971. Hardcover with dustjacket.
212 pages. Concerns 1940's and 50's New York drug scene.
$15.00

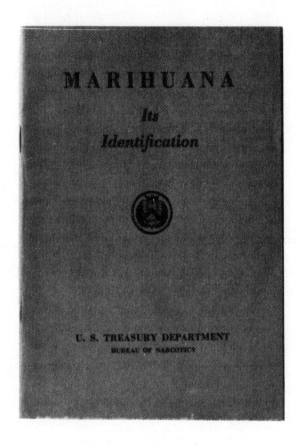

Marihuana—Its Identification
by U. S. Treasury Dept.—Bureau of Narcotics. 1948. Forty
pages with photos. $35.00

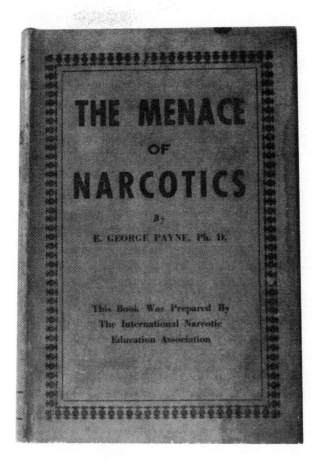

The Menace of Narcotics
by E. George Payne, Ph.D. 1st edition, 1931. Hardcover with dustjacket. 287 pages. $35.00

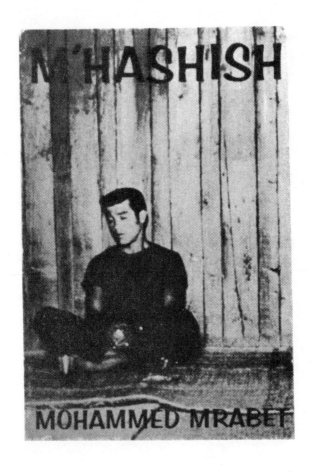

M'Hashish
by Mohammed Mrabet. 3rd printing, 1976. Papercover. $20.00

Musk, Hashish and Blood
by Hector France. Privately printed and undated. 258 pages.
$35.00

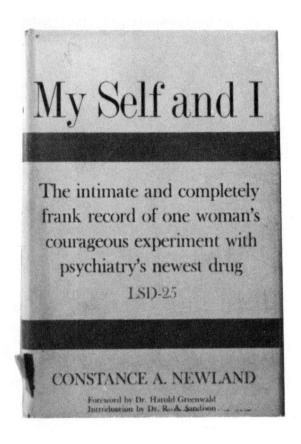

My Self and I
by Constance Newland. 3rd printing, 1962. Hardcover with
dustjacket. 288 pages. $20.00

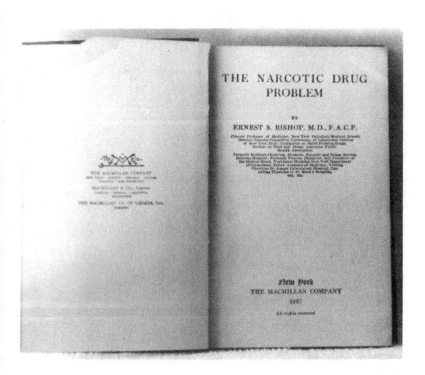

The Narcotic Drug Problem
by Ernest Bishop, M.D. 1921 printing. Hardcover, 165 pages.
$30.00

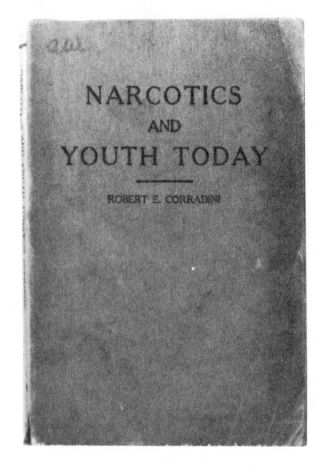

Narcotics and Youth Today
by Robert E. Corradini. 1st edition, 1934. 113 pages with illustrations. $35.00

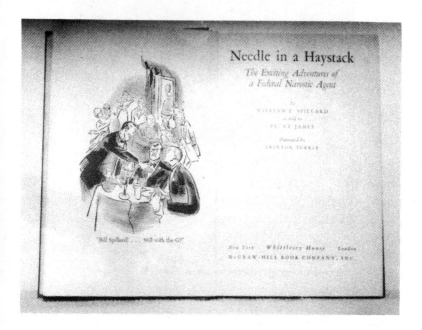

Needle in a Haystack—The Exciting Adventures of a Federal Narcotic Agent

by William Spillard. 1st edition, 1945. Hardcover, 193 pages. $35.00

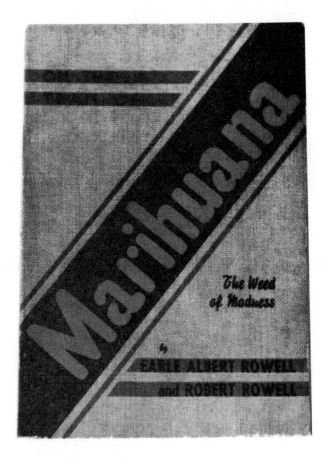

On the Trail of Marihuana—The Weed of Madness
by Earle and Robert Rowell. 1st edition, 1939. Papercover. 96
pages with photos. $60.00

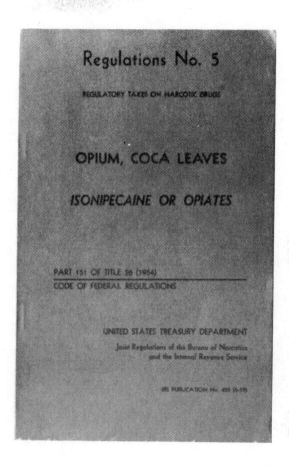

Opium, Coca Leaves, Isonipecaine, or Opiates— Regulation No. 5

by U. S. Treasury Dept. 1959. Papercover, 108 pages. $30.00

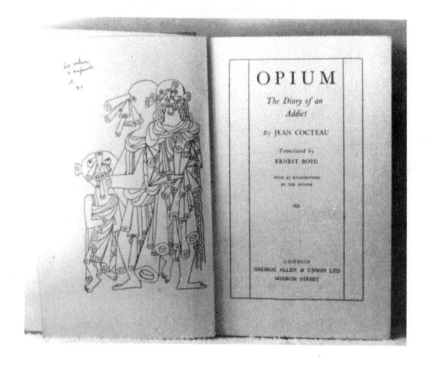

Opium—The Diary of an Addict
by Jean Cocteau. 1st British edition, 1933. Hardcover with illustrations. 187 pages. $50.00

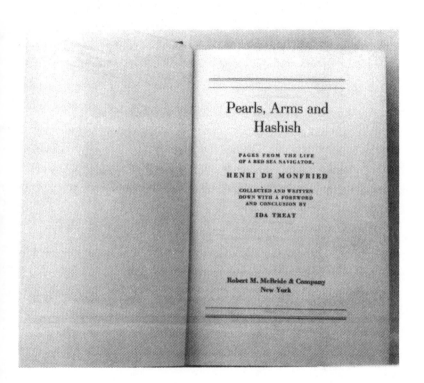

Pearls, Arms and Hashish

by Henri DeMonfried. 1st edition, 1930. Hardcover. 356 pages with photos. $30.00

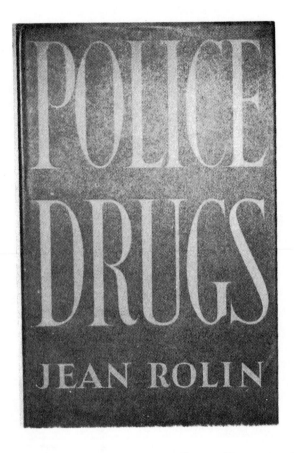

Police Drugs—With an Appendix on Narcoanalysis
by Jean Rolin. 1st edition, 1956. Hardcover with dustjacket. 194
pages. $35.00

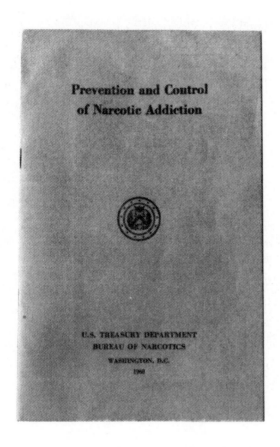

Prevention and Control of Narcotic Addiction
by U. S. Treasury-Bureau of Narcotics. 1960. 32 pages with illustrations. Papercover. $35.00

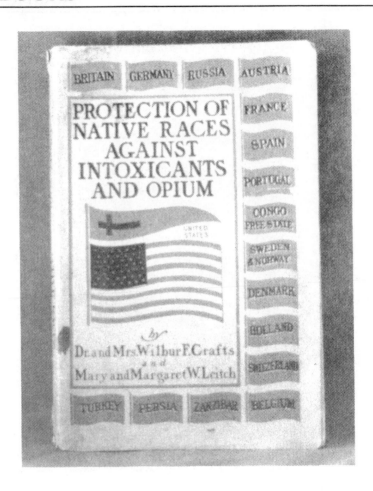

Protection of Native Races Against Intoxicants and Opium
by Crafts and Leitch. 1st edition, 1901. Papercover, 288 pages.
$35.00

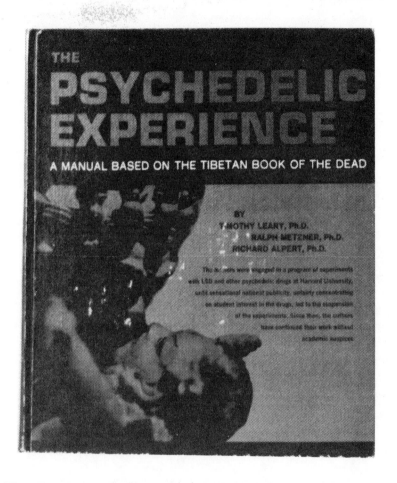

The Psychedelic Experience
by Timothy Leary, Ralph Metzner and Richard Alpert. 3rd printing, 1965. Hardcover, 159 pages. $30.00

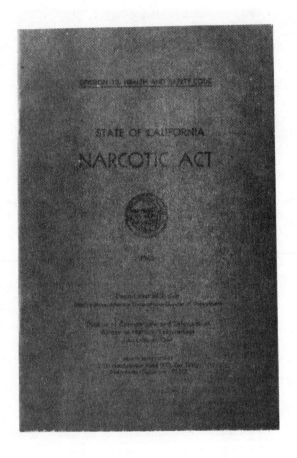

State of California Narcotic Act—1963
Papercover, 50 pages. $30.00

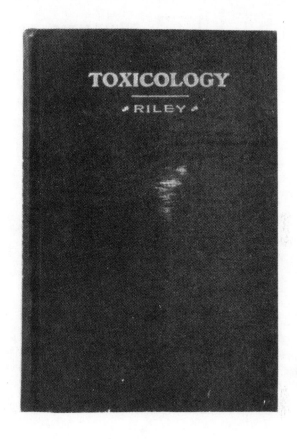

Toxicology
by Cassius Riley, M.D. 2nd edition, 1904. Hardcover, 132
pages. Covers cocaine, opium, morphine, etc. $30.00

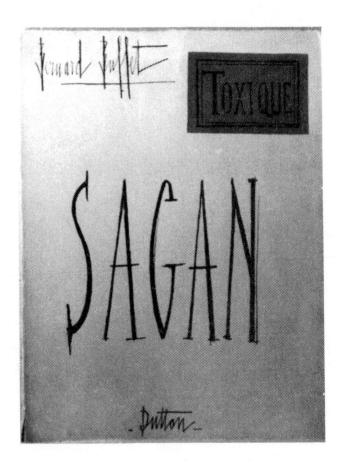

Toxique
by Francoise Sagan. Illustrated by Bernard Buffet. 1st American edition, 1964. Papercover, 72 pages. Concerns Sagans' treatment for morphine addiction. $55.00

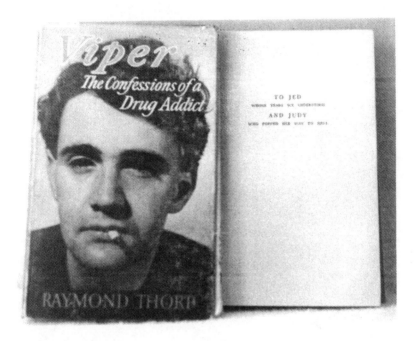

Viper—The Confessions of a Drug Addict
by Raymond Thorp. 1st edition, 1956. Hardcover with
dustjacket. 192 pages. $55.00

26027

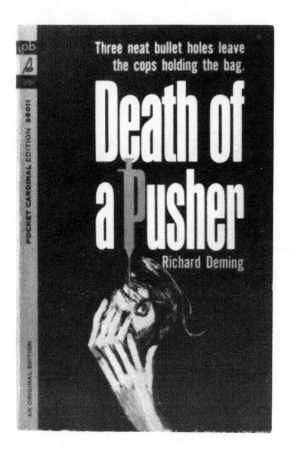

Death of a Pusher
by Richard Deming. 1st printing paperback, 1964. $20.00

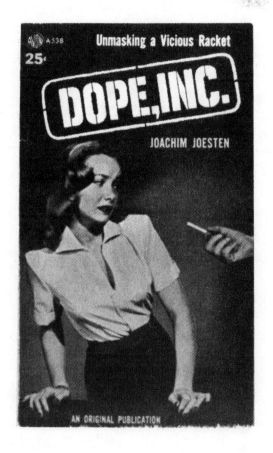

Dope, Inc.
by Joachim Joesten. 1st edition Avon paperback, 1953. $45.00

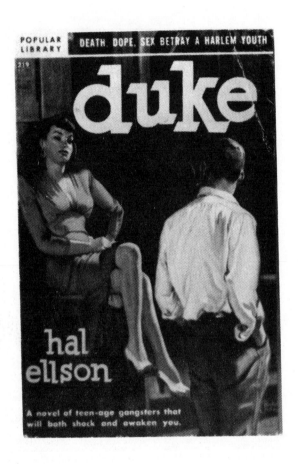

Duke
by Hal Ellson. 6th printing, paperback, 1951. *Death, Dope, Sex Betray a Harlem Youth.* $25.00

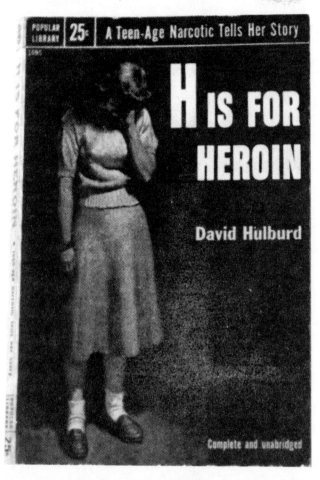

H is for Heroin—A Teenage Narcotic Tells Her Story
by David Hulburd. Popular Library paperback, 1954. $30.00

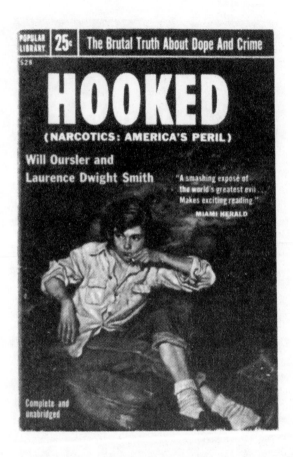

Hooked—Narcotics: America's Peril
by Oursler and Smith. Popular Library paperback, 1953. $45.00

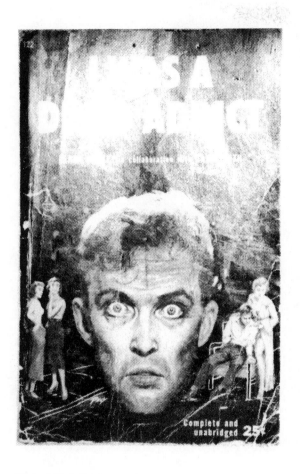

I Was a Drug Addict
by Leroy Street. Pyramid paperback, 1954. $40.00

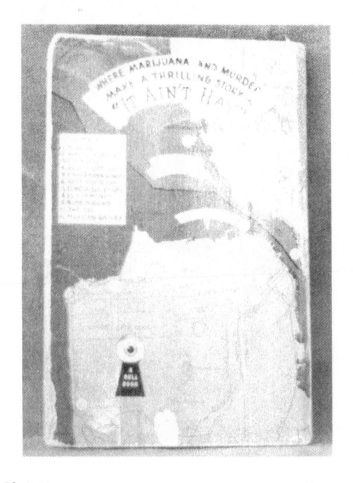

It Ain't Hay
by David Dodge. Dell paperback, 1946. Marijuana and murder
mystery. $40.00

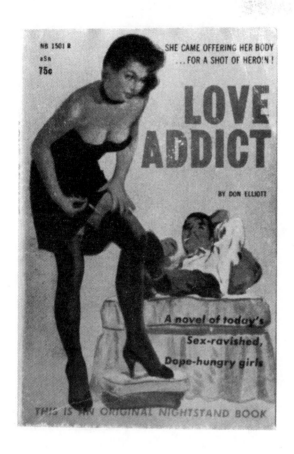

Love Addict
by Don Elliott. 1st edition paperback, 1959. *Offering Her Body for a Shot of Heroin.* $45.00

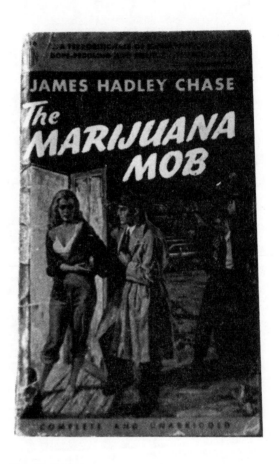

The Marijuana Mob
by James Hadley Chase. Paperback, 1952. $55.00

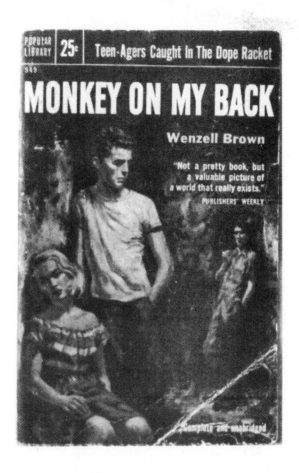

**Monkey On My Back—True Experiences of Teen-Age
Drug Addicts**
by Wenzell Brown. Popular Library paperback, 1954. $45.00

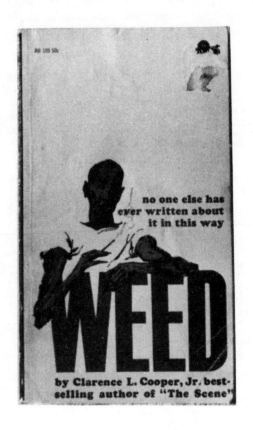

Weed
by Clarence Cooper. 1st edition Regency paperback, 1961. Black ghetto marijuana scene. $30.00

❧ BOTTLES ❧

Most of the following bottles are from the 1880–1920 period.

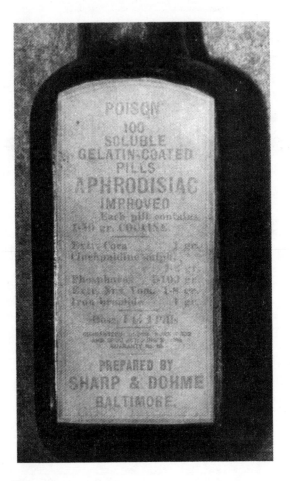

Aphrodisiac
Label lists: *Cocaine 1-50 gr.*, *Extra. Coca l gr.* 3″ tall and corked.
100 pills. Sharpe & Dohme, Baltimore. $100.00

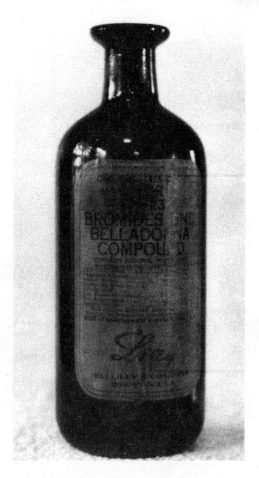

Bromides and Belladonna Compound
Label lists: *Ext. Cannabis U.S.P. 1-8 gr. per oz.* 7 3/4″ tall. Eli
Lilly Co. $110

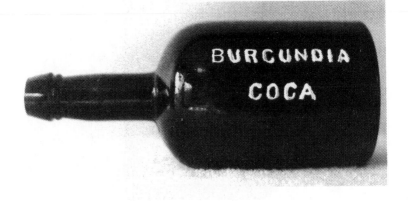

Burgundia Coca
9″ tall, embossed. $100.00

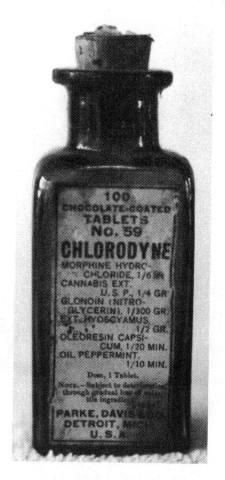

Chlorodyne
Label lists: *Cannabis Ext. U.S.P. 1/4 gr., Morphine Hydrochloride 1/6 gr.* 3½″ tall and corked. Parke, Davis & Co. $110.00

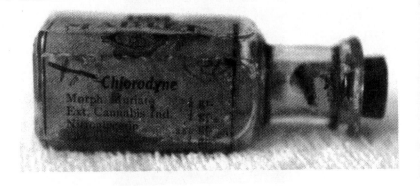

Chlorodyne
Label lists: *Ext. Cannabis Ind. 1/4 gr., Morph. Muriate 1/6 gr.*
3″ tall and corked. Brewer & Co., Worcester, Mass. $110.00

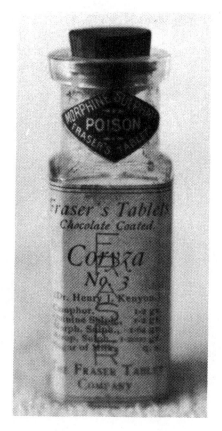

Coryza No. 3
Label lists: *Morphine Sulphate 1-2 gr.* 3″ tall and corked. 100 chocolate coated tablets. Fraser Tablet Co. $25.00

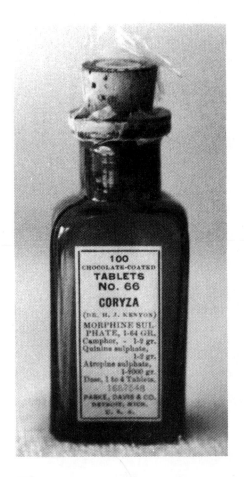

Coryza No. 66
Label lists: *Morphine Sulphate 1-64 gr.* 3″ tall and corked. 100 chocolate coated tablets. Parke, Davis & Co. $25.00

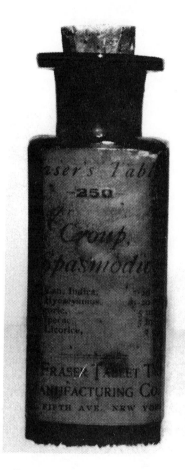

Croup Spasmodic
Lists: *Ext. Can. Indica 1-20 gr., Paregoric 5 min.* 4½″ tall, corked and labeled. Fraser Tablet Co. $110.00

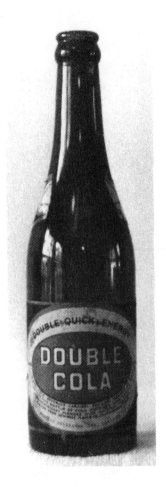

Double Cola
Label lists: *Coca Leaves (Decocanized)*. 9 3/4″ tall. Circa 1940.
$40.00

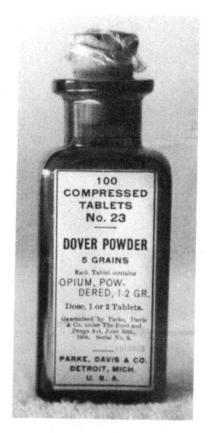

Dover Powder
Label lists: *Opium Powdered 1-2 gr.* 4″ tall and corked. Parke, Davis & Co. Detroit. $25.00

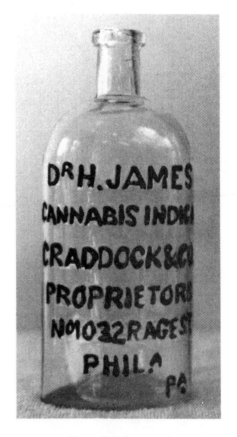

Dr. H. James Cannabis Indica
Craddock & Co. Proprietors, Phila., PA. 7 3/4″ tall, embossed.
$125.00

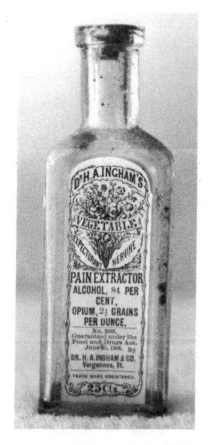

Dr. Ingham's Vegetable Pain Extractor
Label lists: *Opium 2½ grains per oz., Alcohol 84%.* 4 3/4" tall.
$30.00

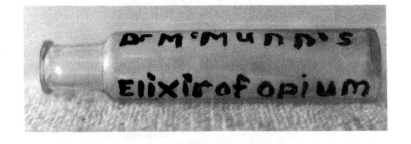

Dr. McMunn's Elixer of Opium
4½" tall and embossed. $20.00

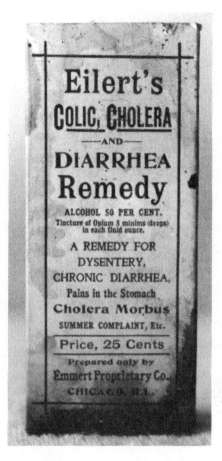

Eilert's Colic, Cholera and Diarrhea Remedy
Box lists: *Tincture of Opium 3 minims.* Emmert Proprietary Co.
4″ tall box with bottle. $25.00

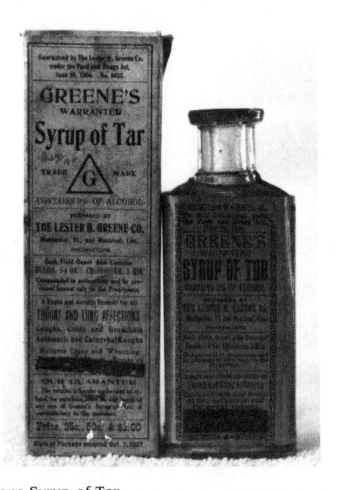

Greens Syrup of Tar
Box and bottle both list: *Heroin 1-4 gr.* 4 3/4″ tall. Green Co., Montpelier, VT. $40.00

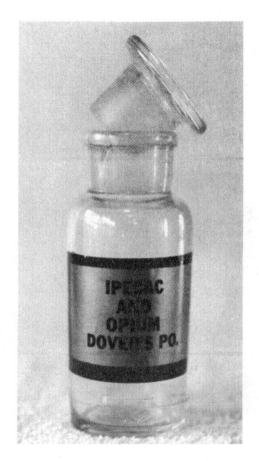

Ipecac and Opium, Dovers PO.
Gold and blue label. 4 3/4″ tall with glass stopper. $70.00

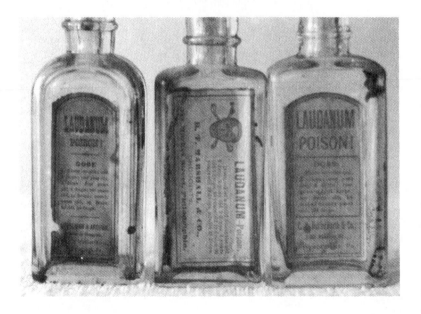

Laudanum
Opium and alcohol preparation. 3 label variations. $25.00 each

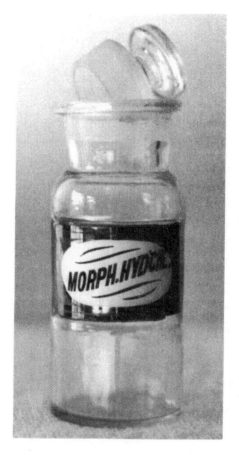

Morph. Hyd'chl.
Red and gold glass label and glass stopper. 5½″ tall. $65.00

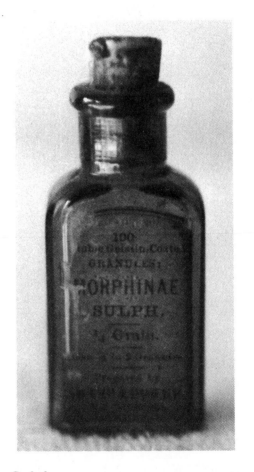

Morphinae Sulph.
2½″ tall and corked. 1/4 gr. Sharpe & Dohme. $25.00

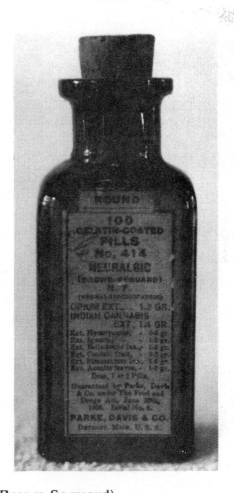

Neuralgic (Brown-Sequard)
Label lists: *Indian Cannabis Ext. 1-4 gr., Opium Ext. 1-2 gr.* 4″
tall and corked. Parke, Davis & Co. $110.00

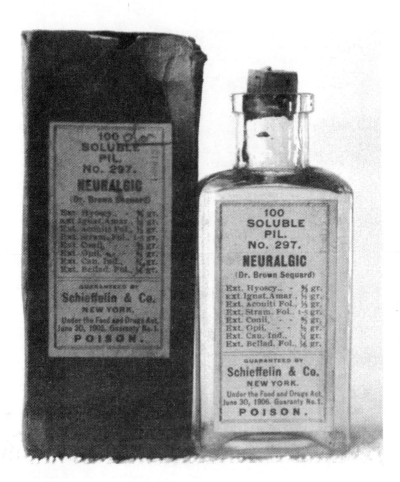

Neuralgic (Dr. Brown Sequard)
Label and box list: *Ext. Can. Ind. 1/4 gr., Ext. Opii 1/2 gr."*
3 3/4" tall and corked. Schieffelin & Co. NY. $120.00

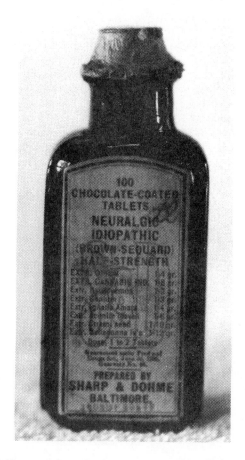

Neuralgic Idiopathic

Label lists: *Extr. Cannabis Ind. 1-8 gr.*, *Extr. Opium 1-4 gr.*
3¼" tall and corked. Sharpe & Dohme, Baltimore. $110.00

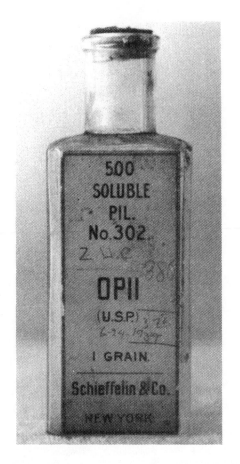

Opii
500 opium pills, 1 grain. Schieffelin & Co., New York. $25.00

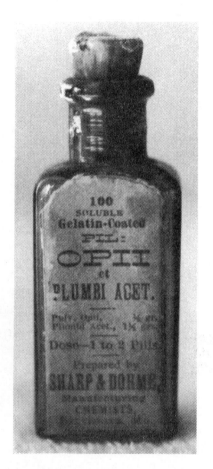

Opii et Plumbi Acet.
Label lists: *Pulv. Opii (opium) 1/2 gr.* 3″ tall and corked. Sharpe
& Dohme. $25.00

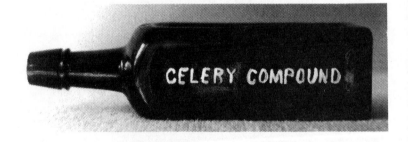

Paine's Celery Compound
Contained coca leaves. 10″ tall and embossed. $15.00

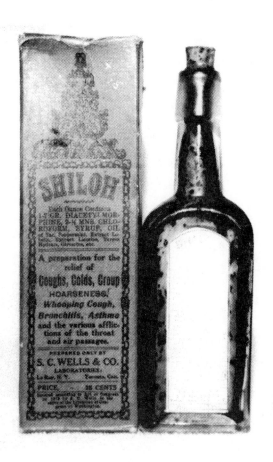

Shiloh
Box and bottle list: *Diacetyl Morphine* (Heroin). 6″ tall. S. C.
Wells & Co., NY. $35.00

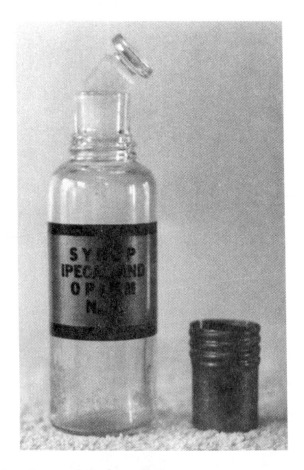

Syrup Ipecac and Opium N.F.
Gold and blue label. 5″ tall with glass stopper and metal screw
on measuring cap. $70.00

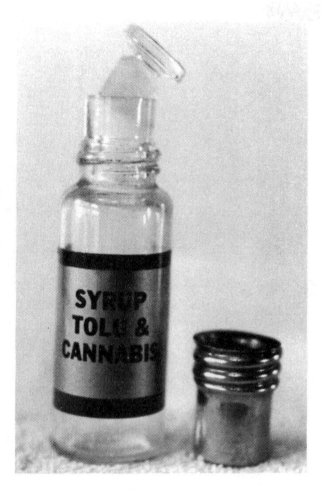

Syrup Tolu & Cannabis
Gold and blue label. 4 3/4″ tall with glass stopper and metal screw on measuring cap. $120.00

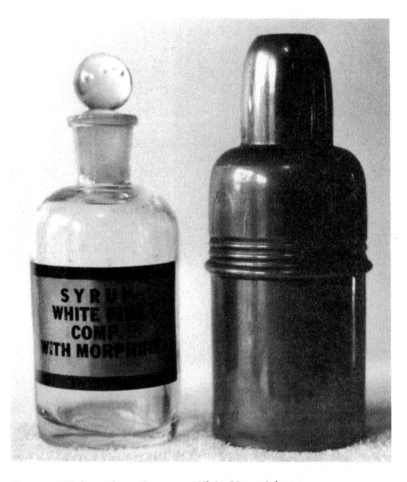

Syrup White Pine Comp. With Morphine
Gold and blue label. 6½" tall with glass stopper and two-piece
metal container stamped, *Germany*. $110.00

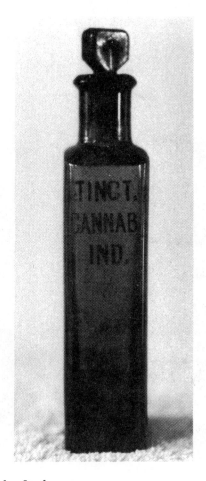

Tinct. Cannab. Ind.
Emerald colored with ribbed sides and glass stopper. 5¼″ tall.
$110.00

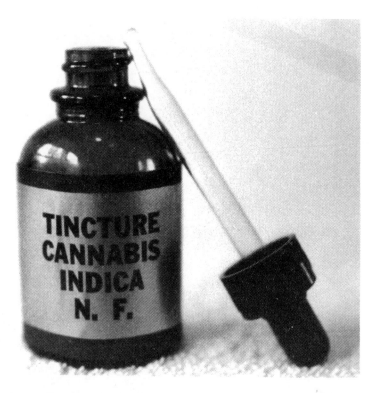

Tincture Cannabis Indica, N.F.
Gold and blue label. 3½" tall with rubber topped glass dropper.
$120.00

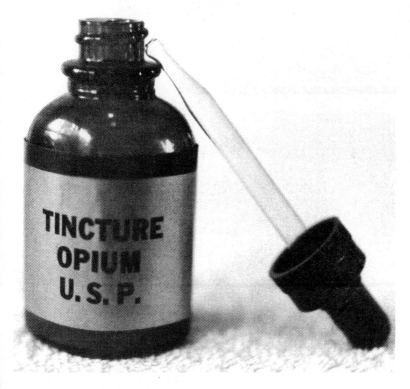

Tincture Opium U.S.P.
Gold and blue label. 3″ tall with rubber-top glass dropper. $70.00

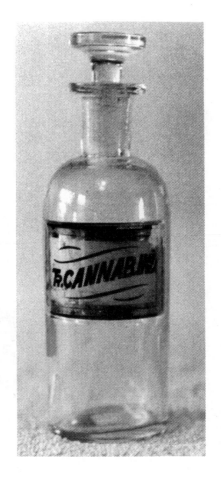

Tr. Cannab. Ind.
6½″ tall with glass label and stopper. $110.00

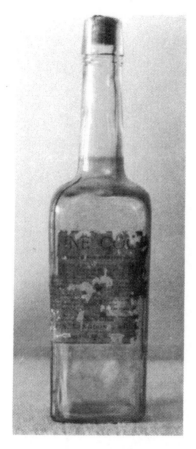

Wine Coca
11″ tall and corked. Label heavily worn. $45.00

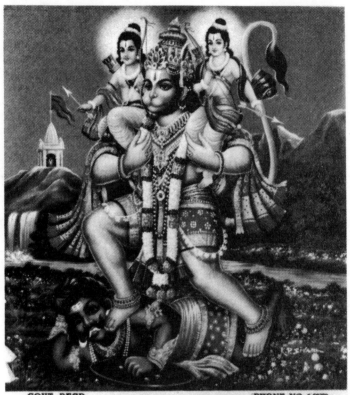

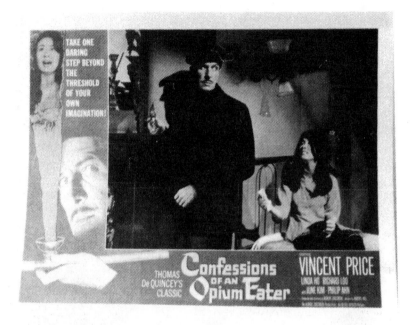

Confessions of an Opium Eater
1962 movie lobby card. Vincent Price. 11" × 14" $25.00

Central Hashish Store
25" × 19" poster. *For Best Nepalese Hashish and Ganja.* From Nepal. $45.00

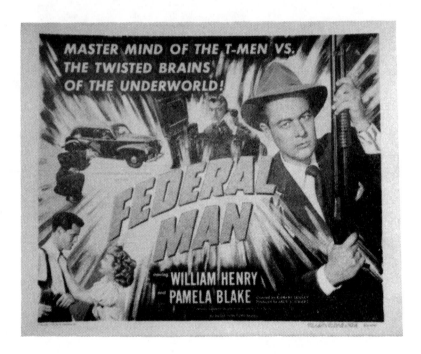

Federal Man
1950 movie lobby card. Movie concerned U.S. narcotics agent
after Mexican and American dope peddlars. 11″ × 14″. $25.00

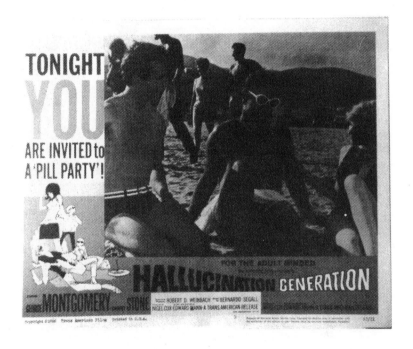

Hallucination Generation
1967 movie lobby card. George Montgomery. 11″ × 14″. $20.00

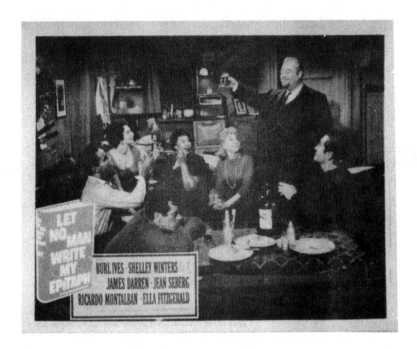

Let No Man Write My Epitaph
1960 movie lobby card. Movie concerned drug addiction. 11″ ×
14″. Burl Ives, Shelly Winters, James Darren. $25.00

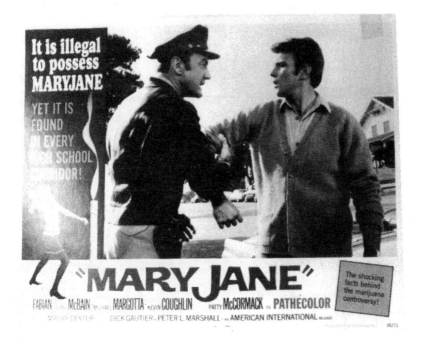

Mary Jane
1968 movie lobby card. Fabian, Dianne McBain. 11″ × 14″.
$30.00

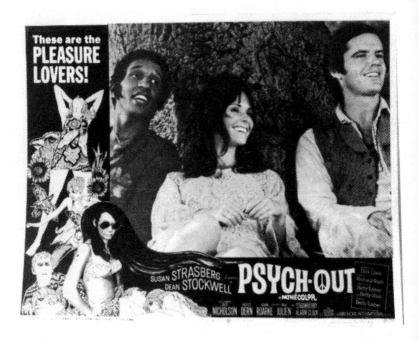

Psych-Out
1968 movie lobby card. Jack Nicholson, Bruce Dern, Susan
Strasberg, Dean Stockwell. 11″ × 14″. $25.00

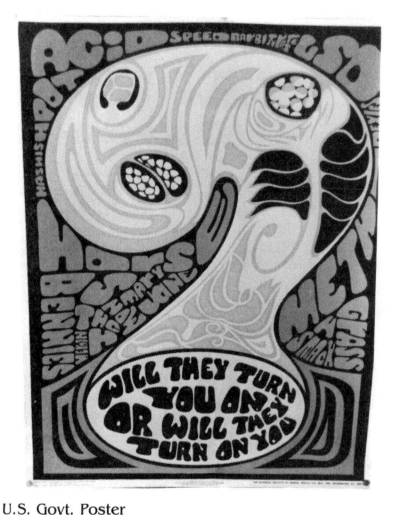

U.S. Govt. Poster
1970 psychedelic poster reads: *Pot, Acid, Speed, Maryjane,
Meth, H—Will They Turn You On, or Turn On You.* 22″ ×
28″. $25.00

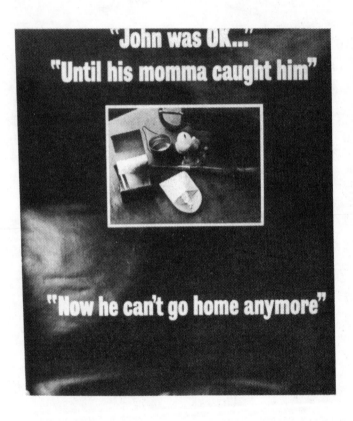

15½ × 17½″ poster, circa 1970. Pictures heroin works. $20.00

MAGAZINES

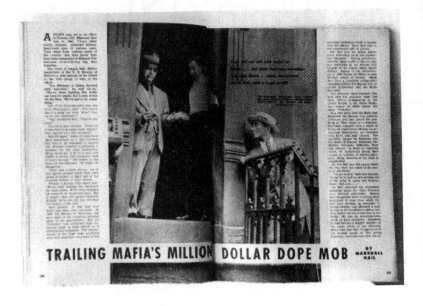

Amazing Detective,
November 1945. Contains article: *Trailing Mafia's Million Dollar Dope Mob.* 8 pages with photos. $25.00

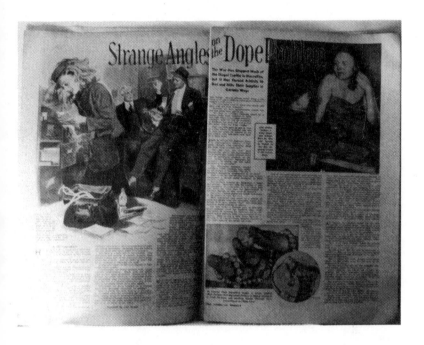

The American Weekly,
July 1945. Contains article: *Strange Angles on the Dope Problem.*
(*A Cokey and his moll robbing a doctor*). Two pages with photos
and illustrations. $35.00

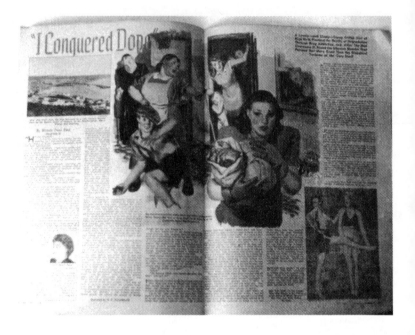

The American Weekly,
July 1946. Contains article: *I Conquered Dope* by actress Brenda
Dean Paul. Two pages with photos and illustrations. $30.00

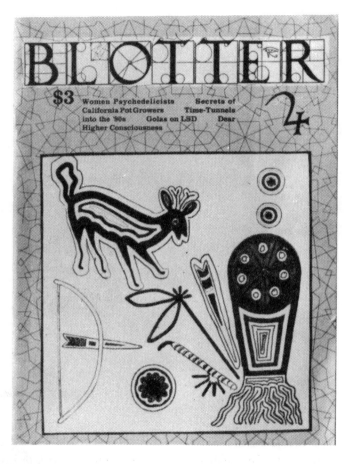

Blotter,
#4 1979. All drug articles. $30.00

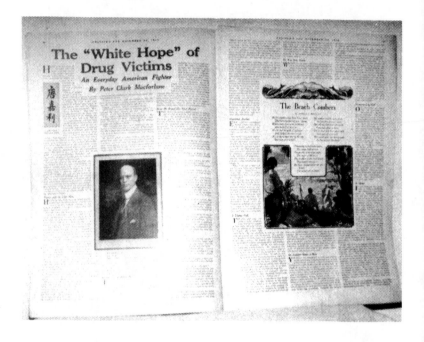

Colliers Magazine,
Nov. 1913. Contains 4-page article with photos: *The White Hope of Drug Victims*. 10½″ × 15″. $30.00

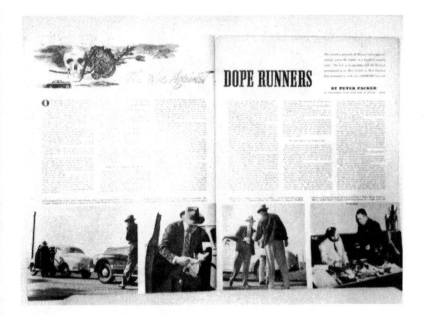

Colliers Magazine,
July 1948. Contains three-page article with photos: *The War Against Dope Runners*. $30.00

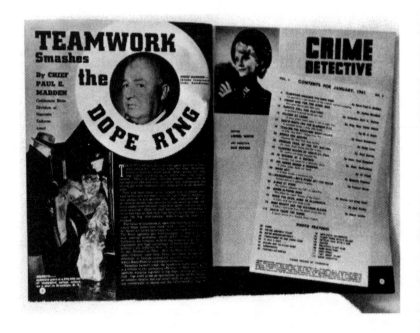

Crime Detective,
1941. Contains article: *Teamwork Smashes the Dope Rings. (25 Tons of Weed Seized in Sacramento.)* Photos. $25.00

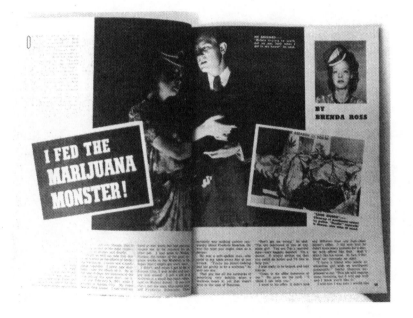

Crime Detective,
1945. Contains article: *I Fed the Marijuana Monster (Vicious Criminals Fatten on the Ruins of Youth.)* 6 pages with photos. $25.00

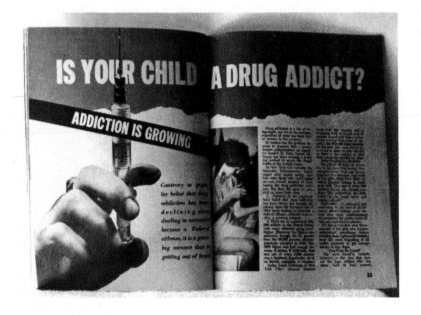

Exclusive,
May 1956. Contains article: *Is Your Child a Drug Addict?* Six
pages with photos. $30.00

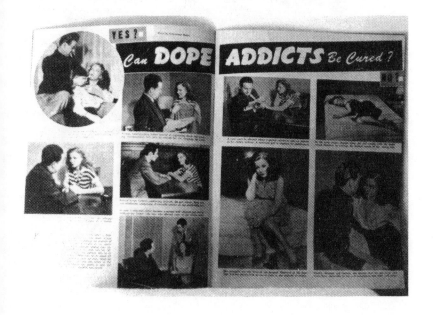

Glance,
June-July 1951. Contains article: *Can a Dope Addict Be Cured?*
(*Will dope destroy our youth?*) Photos. $25.00

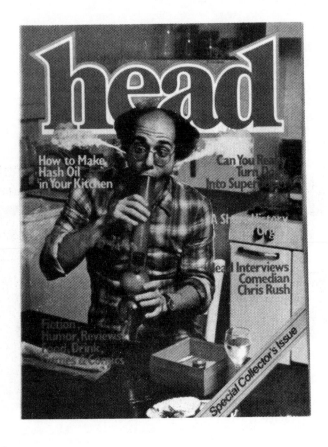

Head,
September 1976. Magazine format. All drug articles. $30.00

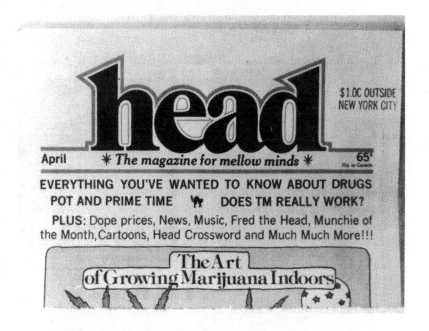

Head—The Magazine for Mellow Minds,
April 1976. Newspaper format. All drug articles. $30.00

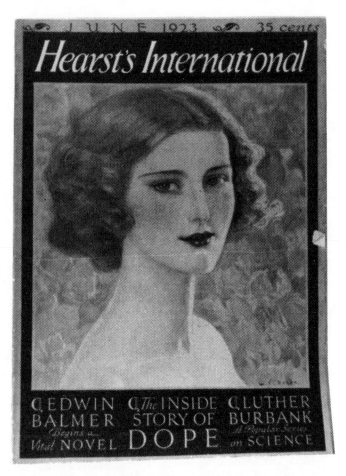

Hearst's International,
June 1923. Cover story: *The Inside Story of Dope in This Country.* Nine pages with photos. $40.00

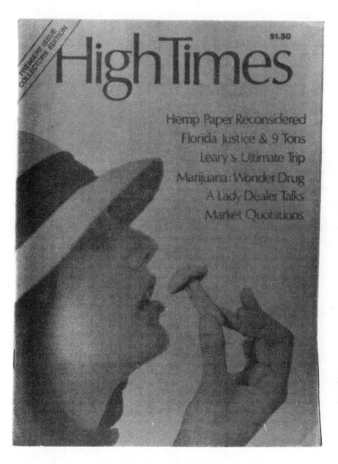

High Times,
Summer 1974. Issue #1. All drug articles. $45.00

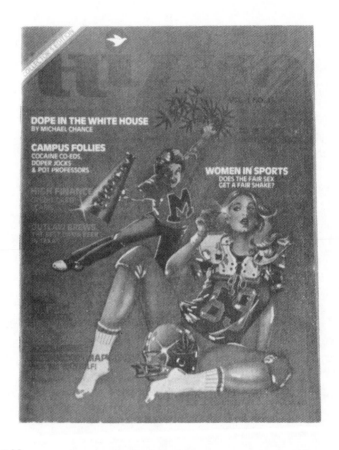

Hi-Life,
December 1978. All drug articles. $30.00

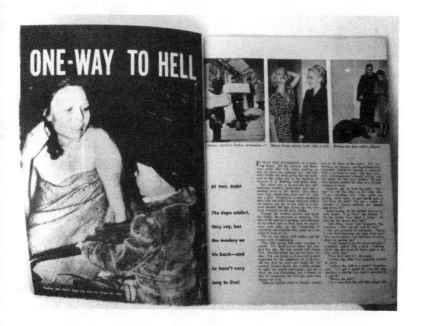

Inside Detective,
November 1950. Contains article: *One-Way To Hell.* (*The dope addict has the monkey on his back*). Five pages with photos. $25.00

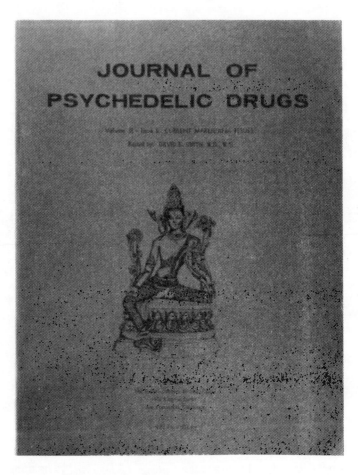

Journal of Psychedelic Drugs,
Fall 1968. Marijuana issue. 166 pages. $25.00

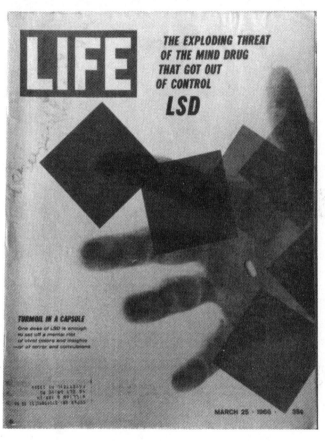

Life,
March 25, 1966. Cover story: *LSD—The Exploding Threat of the Mind Drug That Got Out of Control.* Two articles. Ten pages with photos. $25.00

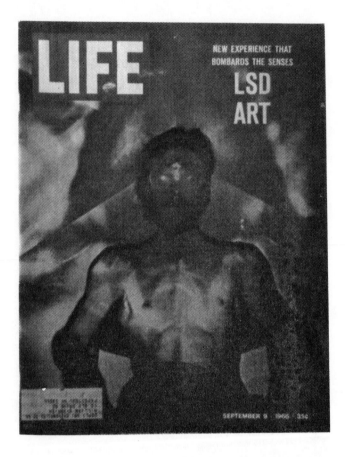

Life,
September 9, 1966. Cover story: *LSD Art.* Nine pages with photos. $25.00

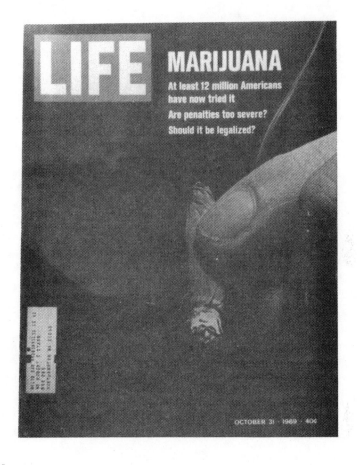

Life,
October 31, 1969. Cover story: *Marijuana—At Least 12 Million Americans Have Now Tried It.* Six pages with photos. $30.00

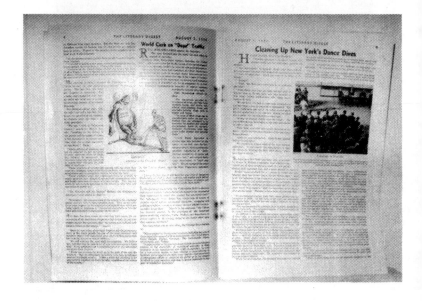

Literary Digest Magazine,
August 1931. Contains ½ page article: *World Curb on Dope Traffic.* $25.00

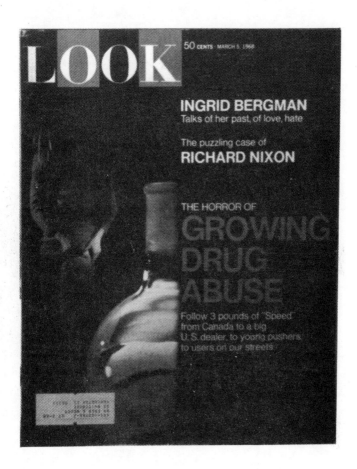

Look,
March 5, 1968. Cover story: *The Horror of Growing Drug Abuse.*
Three articles. Twelve pages with photos. $25.00

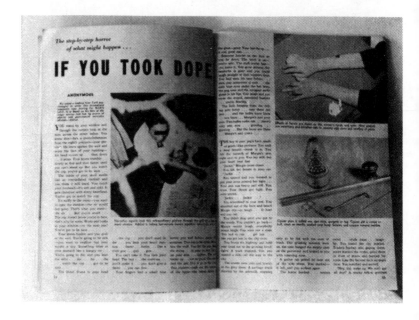

Man's Life,
November 1952. Contains article: *If You Took Dope—The Step by Step Horror of What Might Happen.* Seven pages with photos. $30.00

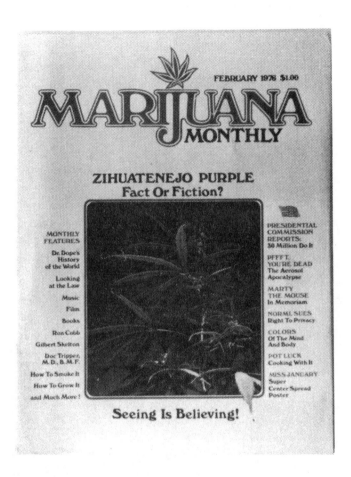

Marijuana Monthly,
February 1976. All drug articles. $30.00

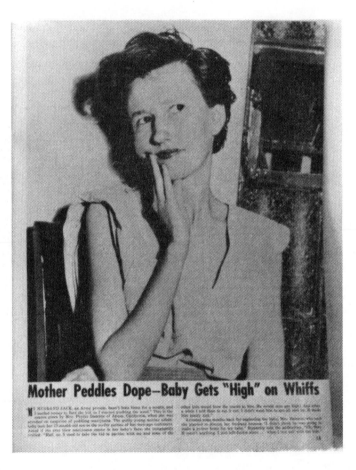

Now,
February 1955. Contains one full-page picture of *Mother Peddles Dope—Baby Gets High on Whiffs*. $25.00

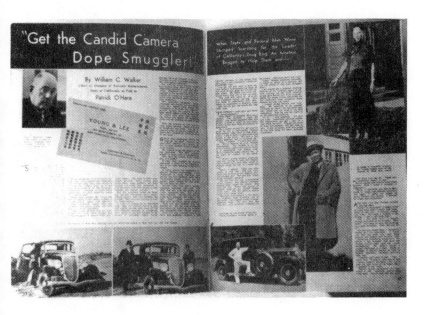

Official Detective,
December 1937. Contains article: *Get the Candid Camera Dope Smuggler.* Six pages with photos. $25.00

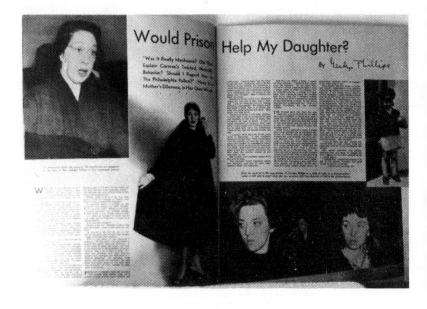

Official Detective,
July 1956. Contains article: *Would Prison Help My Daughter?*
(*Was it really marihuana?*) Five pages with photos. $25.00

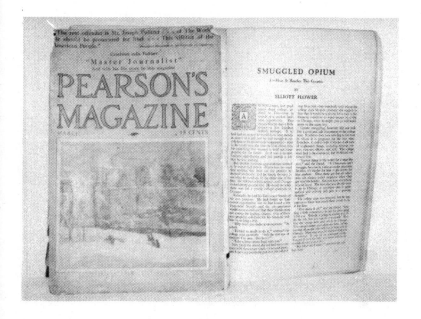

Pearson's Magazine,
March 1909. Contains seven-page article: *Smuggled Opium—How It Reaches This Country.* $30.00

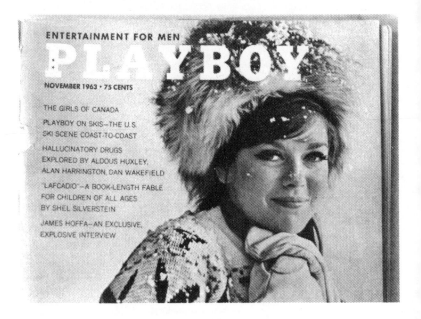

Playboy,
November 1963. Cover story: *Hallucinatory Drugs Explored by Aldous Huxley, Alan Harrington, Dan Wakefield.* Three articles with photos. $25.00

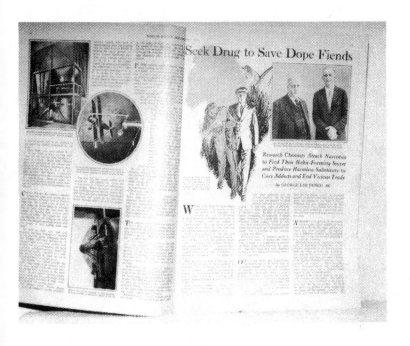

Popular Science Monthly Magazine,
May 1931. Contains three-page article with photos: *Seek Drug to Save Dope Fiends.* $25.00

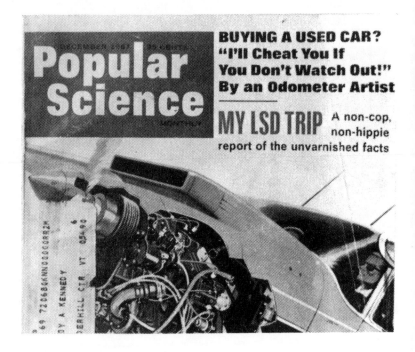

Popular Science,
December 1967. Cover story: *My LSD Trip—A Non-Cop, Non-Hippie Report of the Unvarnished Facts.* Eight pages. $25.00

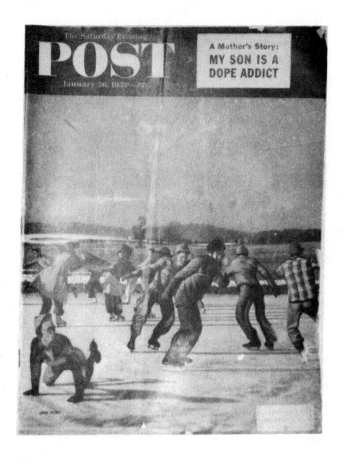

Post Magazine,
January 1952. Seven-page cover story with photos: *My Son is a Dope Addict.* $25.00

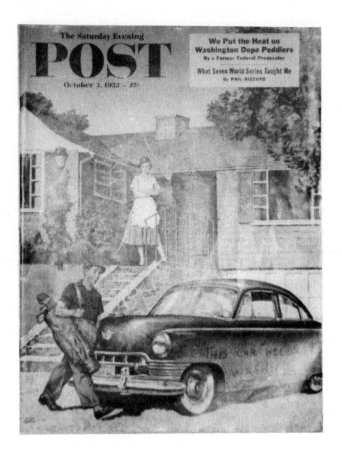

Post Magazine,
October 1953. Five page cover story with photos: *We Put the Heat on Washington Dope Peddlers.* $25.00

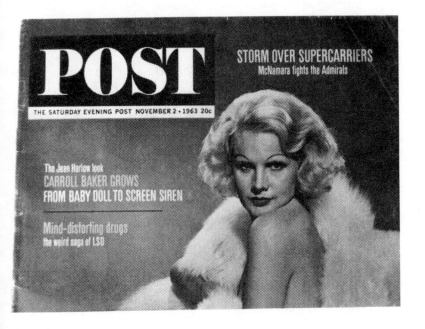

Post,
November 2, 1963. Cover story: *Mind-Distorting Drugs—The Weird Saga of LSD.* Seven pages with photos. $25.00

Post,
August 12, 1967. Cover story: *The Newly Discovered Dangers of LSD—To the Mind, Body and Unborn.* Five pages with photos. $25.00

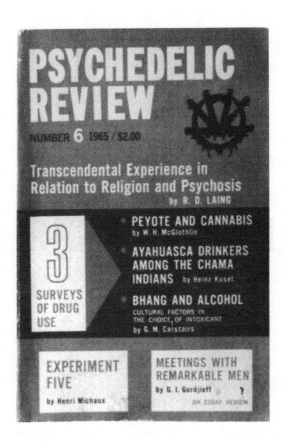

Psychedelic Review,
1965. Issue #6. All drug articles. $25.00

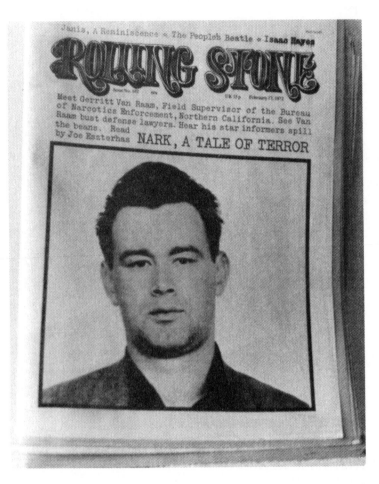

Rolling Stone,
February 17, 1972. Contains cover article: *Nark, A Tale of Terror.* Nine pages with photos. $15.00

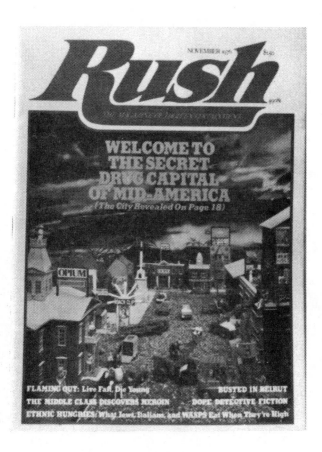

Rush—The Magazine of High Entertainment,
November 1976. All drug articles. $30.00

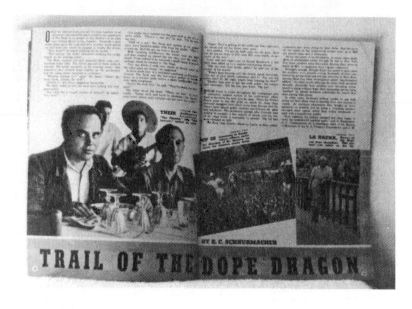

Sensation,
December 1943. Contains article: *Trail of the Dope Dragon—U. S. Agents Make It Hot for Dope Smugglers.* Concerns U.S.-Mexico Dope Smuggling. Seven pages with photos. $20.00

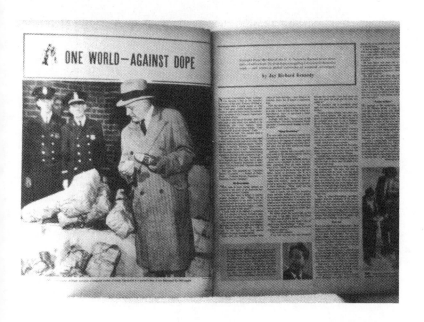

This Week,
March 1948. Contains article: *One World Against Dope.* Four
pages with photos. $25.00

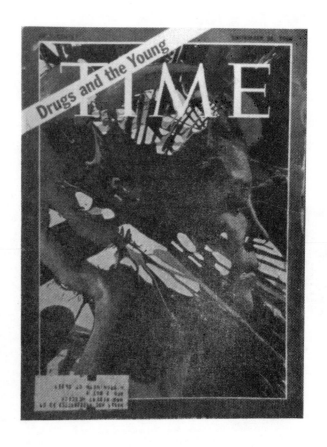

Time,
September 26, 1972. Cover story: *Drugs and the Young.* Eight pages with photos. $20.00

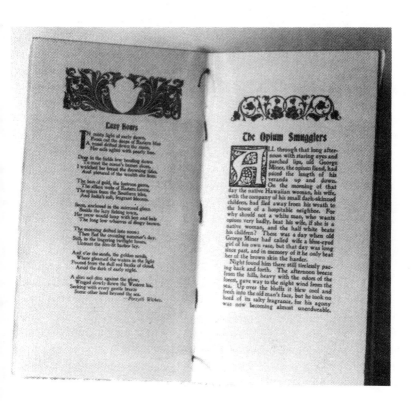

Yale Courant,
circa 1898. Contains article: *The Opium Smugglers*. Six pages.
$40.00

AMERICAN ENSLAVEMENT TO DRUGS

NATIVE-BORN AMERICANS are said to possess less self-control than foreigners in this country in the use of narcotic drugs. It is no matter for self-congratulation that of all white races, and indeed of all races, except the yellow, where the use of opium and hashish is deeply established, we are the greatest drug addicts in the world. This is not a mere supposition, but a fact established on the testimony of a competent committee appointed by the Secretary of the Treasury to make a national investigation of the drug habit. Their report will shortly be made public, but a preliminary abstract appears in the New York Times. The writer here expects that, in view of these revelations and the recent ones respecting the prevalence of the use of drugs in New York, some measures will be coupled with the prohibition act to counteract the use of these narcotic stimulants. Much evidence is said to have been gathered by the committee in various parts of the country on the alternative drug-stimulation after prohibition has been put into effect, but this is admitted to be too conflicting to furnish a clear prognosis. We see that—

"In some parts of the country, notably in large cities like New York, Philadelphia, and Pittsburg, the liquor and drug habits were found to be gathering more victims side by side. On the other hand, in some parts of the country where prohibition had gone into effect—in sections of Kentucky, Albama, and Texas, for example—extensive use of paregoric and similar compounds containing morphin was discovered. In one Kentucky dry county two per cent. of the inhabitants, it was estimated, are

should be given by the [...]
regulated by them.

"General hospitals are [...] are inadequate. In every [...] law is enforced, deaths of [...] sult unless there were an [...] cocain habit can be stop[...] ease, experts say, but no [...] these are abruptly taken [...] with foaming at the mo[...] usually follows."

The effect of prohibit[...] stimulants to excess is [...] problem that will follow t[...]

"Unless the States coo[...] at present, the machine[...] drink from turning to d[...] that prohibition has had [...] is a question debated wit[...] statistics it is an open [...] figures from those who ar[...] growth in drug victims. [...] is that the drug evil is a[...] secret dealing because of [...] that an army of governm[...] to what an extent the pra[...]

"In seeking to keep the [...] the prohibition amendm[...] Washington will seek [...] There is no doubt that [...] tionally caused many to [...] Morphin given with go[...] to the patient's later sta[...] few physicians, it is assert[...]

American Enslavement to Drugs.
One-page article from *Literary Digest*, April 1919. $25.00

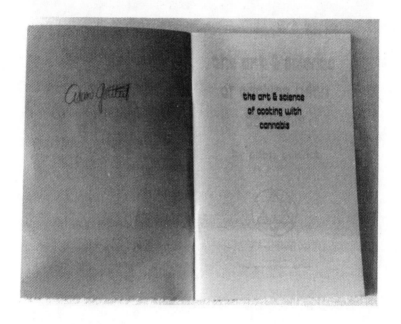

The Art and Science of Cooking with Cannabis
by Adam Gottlieb. Hand-signed by author. 1st edition, 1974. 77
pages. $30.00

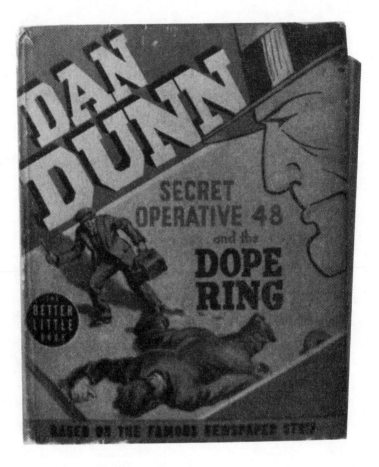

Dan Dunn—Secret Operative 48 and the Dope Ring
by Norman Marsh. *Big Little Book*, 3½″ × 4½″. 1940. 420
pages with illustrations. $35.00

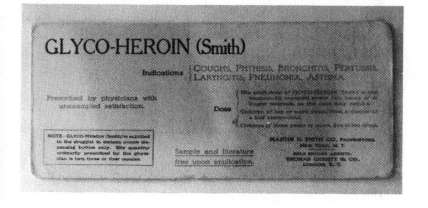

Glyco-Heroin
4″ × 9″ advertising blotter. Smith Co., circa 1910. $25.00

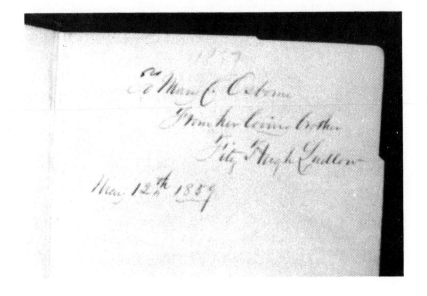

The Hasheesh Eater
by Fitz Hugh Ludlow. Enscribed by author: *To Mary C. Osborne, from her loving brother, Fitz Hugh Ludlow—May 12, 1859.* 1st edition, 1857. Hardcover, 371 pages. $200.00

HOW THE OPIUM-HABIT IS ACQUIRED.

By VIRGIL G. EATON.

I AM not one of the persons who raise a great cry about the evils of the "opium-habit." I have no doubt that the continued use of narcotics, whether they be tobacco or opium, is injurious to the nervous system; but I also firmly believe that the recuperative powers of the body are such that they can largely overcome any harmful results coming from the regular use of these substances. For instance, I know a stone-cutter who resides at Cape Elizabeth, Me., who for the past twenty years has used twenty cents' worth of black "navy plug" tobacco every day. He is a large, vigorous man, weighing over two hundred pounds. His appetite is good; he sleeps well, and, save for a little heart disturbance caused by overstimulation, he is perfectly healthy, and is likely to live until he is fourscore. He is now fifty-one years of age, and he assures me he has used tobacco since he was fourteen, and never had a fit of "swearing off" in his life. A peculiar and, I should say, a rather troublesome habit of his, is to go to bed every night with a big "quid" of hard "plug" tobacco between

* The writer will gratefully acknowledge the receipt of additional myths of similar character to those here given, with a view to subsequent fuller treatment of the subject. It will be of service if considerable detail be given in regard to the geographical or social boundaries of the superstition, and if the latter be stated as explicitly as possible. (Address Mrs. Fanny D. Bergen, 17 Arlington St., North Cambridge, Mass.)

How the Opium Habit is Acquired
Ten page article from *The Popular Science Monthly*, 1888.
$30.00

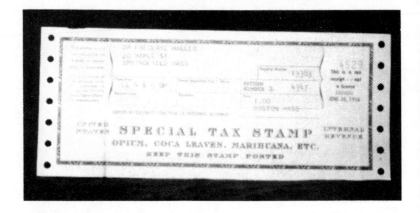

I.R.S. Special Tax Stamp—*Opium, Coca Leaves, Marihuana, Etc.*
1956. 8½" × 3½". $25.00

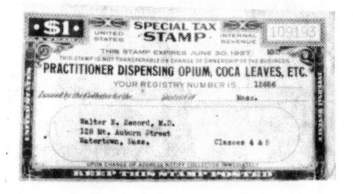

I.R.S. Special Tax Stamp—*Practitioner Dispensing Opium, Coca Leaves, Etc.*
1937. 6½" × 3½". $20.00

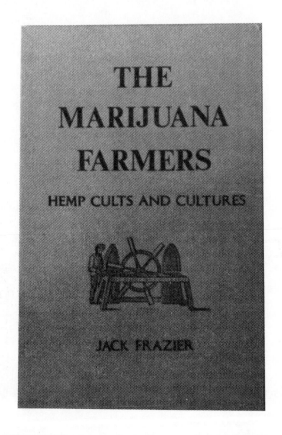

The Marijuana Farmers
by Jack Frazier. Hand-signed by author. 1974. 135 pages. $30.00

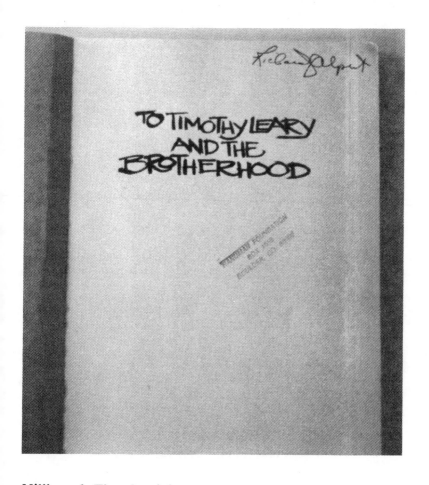

Millbrook Thanksgiving
by Walter Schneider. Hand-signed by Richard Alpert (Ram Dass). 1971 edition of 3,000 copies. $50.00

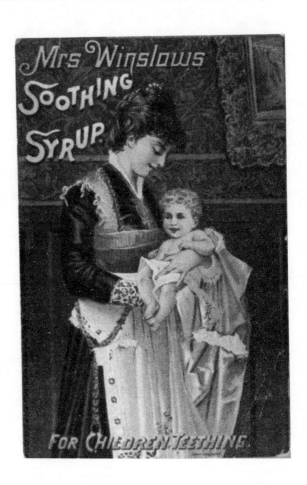

Mrs. Winslow's Soothing Syrup
3½″ × 5″ advertising tradecard. A morphine product. 1888.
$7.00

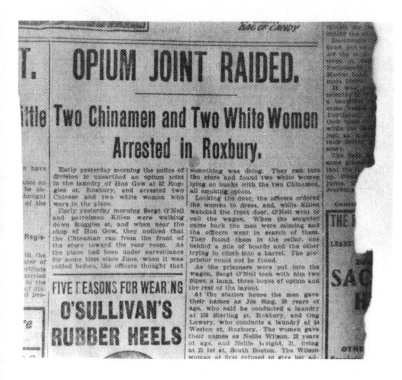

Opium Joint Raided—Two Chinamen and Two White Women Arrested
Two-column story from 1903 Boston Globe newspaper. $25.00

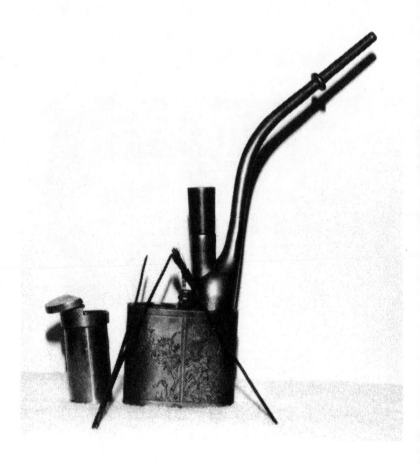

Opium Smoking Set
Complete layout contains 10″ tall pipe, two bowls, tweezers, cleaning brush and hinged brass opium container. Engraved floral design with Chinese characters. Circa 1880. $150.00

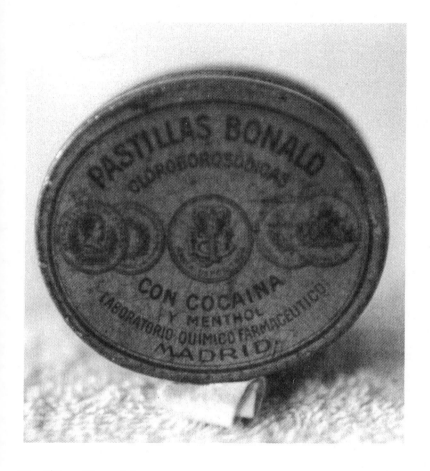

Pastillas Bonald
2¼" × 1¾" × 1" cocaine lozenge tin. Madrid. $100.00

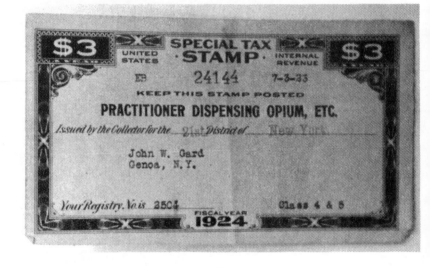

Practitioner Dispensing Opium, Etc.
Special U.S. IRS Tax Stamp. 1923. 3½″ × 6½″. $15.00

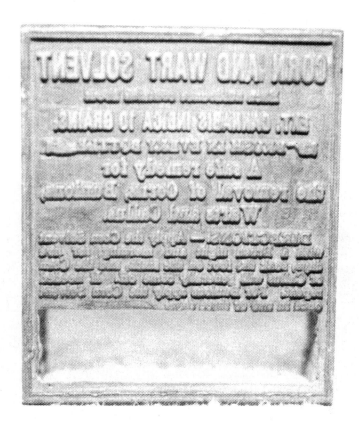

Printers Block
2½" × 2" × 1" wood block reads: *Corn and Wart Remover–Ext. Cannabis Indica 10 Grains,* etc. $60.00

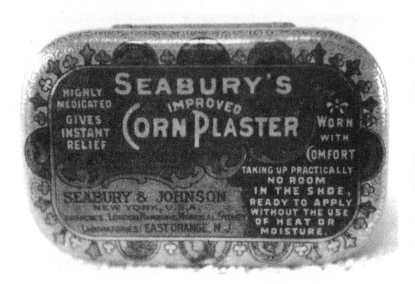

Seabury Corn Plaster
3″ × 2″ red, blue and gold tin reads: *Contains 24 Grains Extract Cannabis.* $65.00

Treasury Dept. Coca Leaves, Opium
Order form, 1936 series. 8½″ × 11″. $15.00

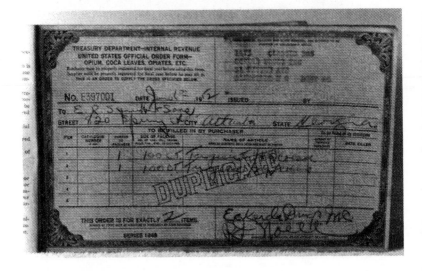

Treasury Dept. Coca Leaves, Opium
Order book with nine forms. 7¾″ × 5″. 1948 series. $20.00

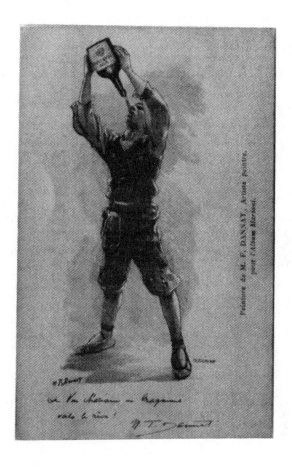

Vin Mariani Coca Wine
Advertising postcard. Circa 1900. $40.00

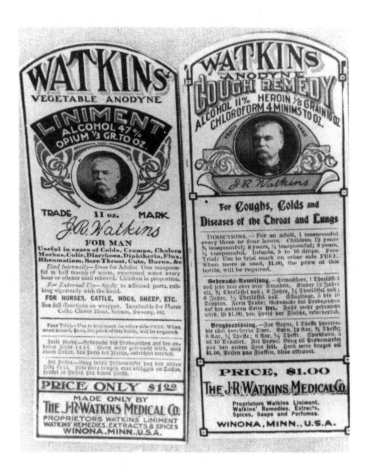

Watkins Products

Two labels, one listing: *Opium ⅓ gr. to oz.*; other listing: *Heroin ⅛ Grain to oz.* Opium label $20.00; Heroin label $30.00

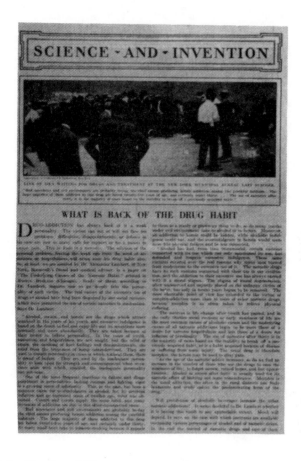

What Is Back of The Drug Habit
Two-page article with photos from *Literary Digest*, 1920. $30.00

~§ PAPER ~ ADVERTISING

The following are turn of the century magazine and newspaper advertisements.

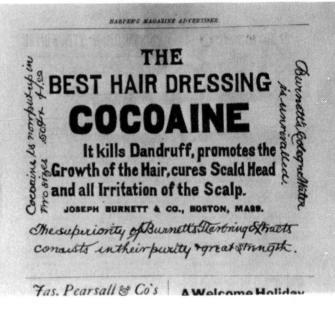

Cocoaine
One-half page from 1896 Harpers Magazine. Did not contain coca or cocaine. $20.00

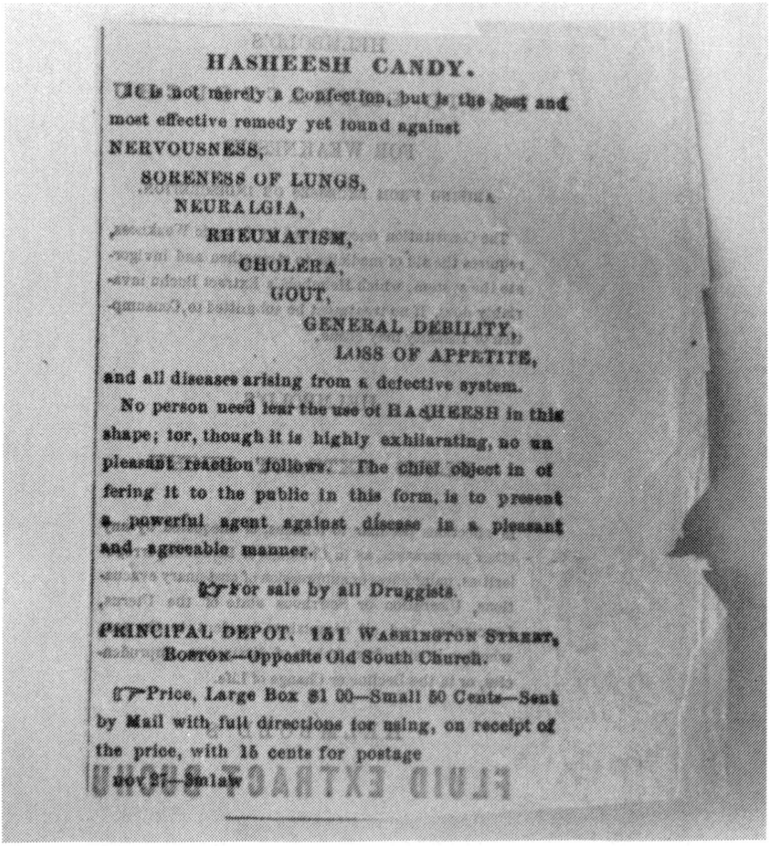

HASHEESH CANDY.

This is not merely a Confection, but is the best and most effective remedy yet found against

NERVOUSNESS,

SORENESS OF LUNGS,

NEURALGIA,

RHEUMATISM,

CHOLERA,

GOUT,

GENERAL DEBILITY,

LOSS OF APPETITE,

and all diseases arising from a defective system.

No person need fear the use of HASHEESH in this shape; for, though it is highly exhilarating, no unpleasant reaction follows. The chief object in offering it to the public in this form, is to present a powerful agent against disease in a pleasant and agreeable manner.

For sale by all Druggists.

PRINCIPAL DEPOT, 151 WASHINGTON STREET, BOSTON—Opposite Old South Church.

Price, Large Box $1 00—Small 50 Cents—Sent by Mail with full directions for using, on receipt of the price, with 15 cents for postage

nov 21—3mlaw

Hasheesh Candy

1866 newspaper ad. 3¾″ × 3¼″. $30.00

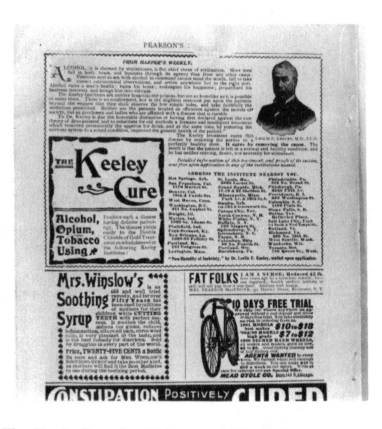

The Keely Cure for Opium and Alcohol,
and below it, ad for *Mrs. Winslow's Soothing Syrup* (Morphine).
1897. 4½″ × 6″. $25.00

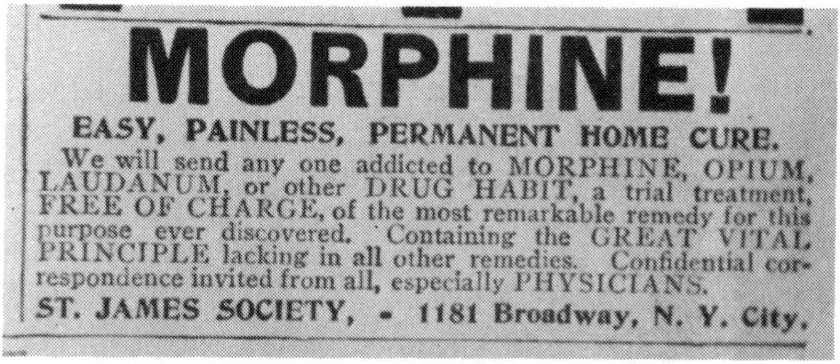

Morphine Home Cure
Munsey's Magazine, 1898. 3½″ × 1″. $20.00

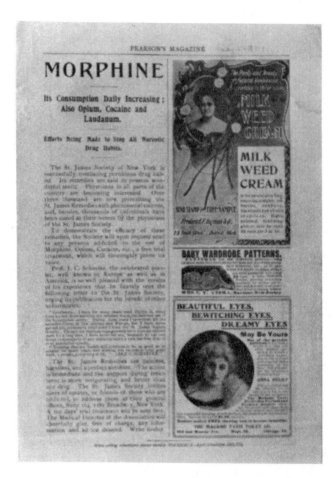

Morphine: Its Consumption Daily Increasing—Also Opium, Cocaine and Laudanum

Cure Advertisement. One-half page. Pearson's Magazine, 1901. $25.00

At the International Medical Congress, lately held in Washington, D. C.

RESTORATIVE WINE OF COCA. The majority of the three thousand delegates tested our Restorative Wine of Coca, and were unanimous in pronouncing it the most palatable and high-class preparation of Coca they had yet examined. **Read the following, from Prof. Semmola:**

WASHINGTON, Sept. 9, 1887.

Having tested and made repeated examinations of the Wine of Coca manufactured by Messrs. Thurber, Whyland & Co., I hereby certify that this preparation is most excellent as a restorative in all cases of general debility of the nervous system, especially in disorders arising from excessive intellectual strain, or other causes producing mental weakness. I also consider this Wine invaluable for the purpose of renewing lost vitality in constitutions enfeebled by prolonged illness, particularly in cases of convalescence from malignant fevers.—**M. Semmola, M. D.**, Prof. of Experimental Pharmacy and Clinical Therapeutics, University of Naples, Italy.

COCANIZED BEEF, WINE, AND IRON. They also pronounce our Cocanized Beef, Wine, and Iron the most palatable and attractive preparation of Beef, Wine, and Iron they had ever seen, and were loud in their praises of it. Physicians cheerfully furnished with samples.

THURBER, WHYLAND & CO. New-York.

Restorative Wine of Coca, and *Cocanized Beef, Wine and Iron*

1888 newspaper ad. Thurber, Whyland & Co., New York. 4″ × 7″. $25.00

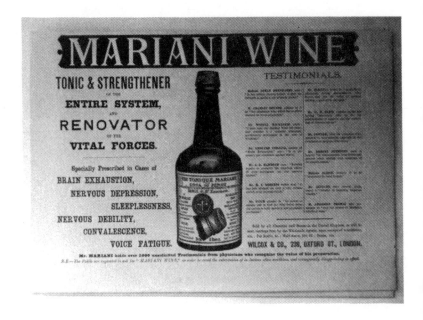

Vin Mariani Coca Wine
From the *Illustrated London News*, 1892. Testimonials by Sarah Bernhardt, Charles Gounod, etc. 11½″ × 16″. $20.00

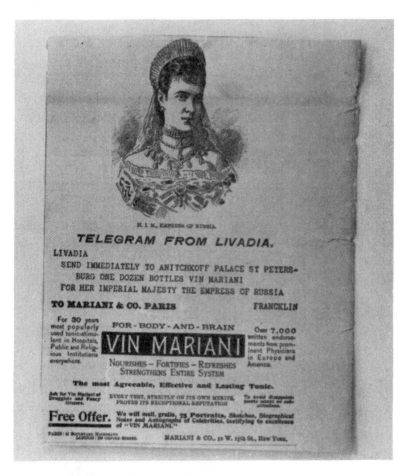

Vin Mariani Coca Wine
Depicting telegram from Empress of Russia requesting Vin
Mariani. 1898. 8½″ × 11″. $25.00

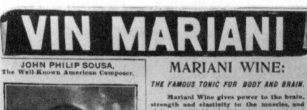

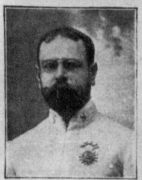

JOHN PHILIP SOUSA,
The Well-Known American Composer.

JOHN PHILIP SOUSA WRITES:
When worn out, I find nothing so helpful as a glass of Vin Mariani. To brain
workers and those who expend a great
deal of nervous force, it is invaluable.
JOHN PHILIP SOUSA.

MARIANI WINE:

THE FAMOUS TONIC FOR BODY AND BRAIN.

Mariani Wine gives power to the brain,
strength and elasticity to the muscles, and
richness to the blood. It is a promoter of good
health and longevity.

Mariani Wine is indorsed by more than
8,000 American physicians. It is specially
indicated for General Debility, Overwork,
Profound Depression and Exhaustion, Throat
and Lung Diseases, Consumption and Malaria.

Mariani Wine is invaluable for over-
worked men, delicate women, and sickly
children. It soothes, strengthens and sustains
the system, and braces body and brain.

When the Grip (influenza) was epidemic
in Europe as also in this country, the Medical
Profession relied upon the tonic properties of
Vin Mariani. It was given as a preventive and
also in convalescence to build up the system
and to avoid the many disagreeable after ef-
fects so common with this dreaded disease.

To those who will kindly write to MARIANI
& CO., 52 West 15th Street, New York City, will be
sent, free, book containing portraits with indorse-
ments of Emperors, Empress, Princes, Cardinals,
Archbishops and other interesting matter. Mention
this publication.

Paris—41 Boulevard Haussmann ; London—83 Morti-
mer Street ; Montreal—28-30 Hospital Street.

Vin Mariani Coca Wine

John Philip Sousa testimonial. 1898. 4¾″ × 4½″. $25.00

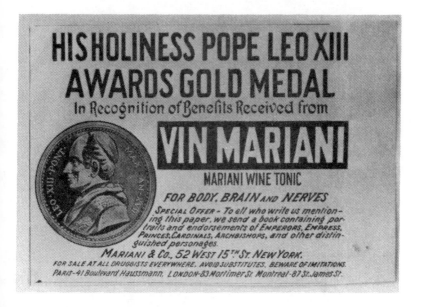

Vin Mariani Coca Wine
Pope Leo XIII Awards Gold Medal to Vin Mariani. 1899. 5¾"
× 3¾". $25.00

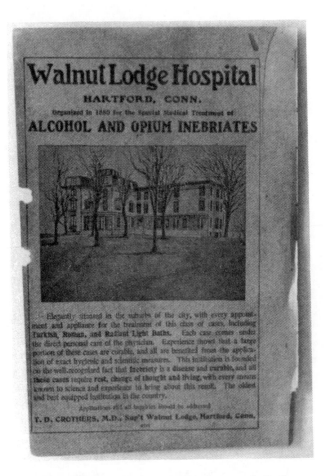

Walnut Lodge Hospital for Alcohol and Opium
Inebriates
Hartford, CT. 1906. 5″ × 7½″. $25.00

❧ POSTCARDS ❧

The following postcards are all from the early 1900's.

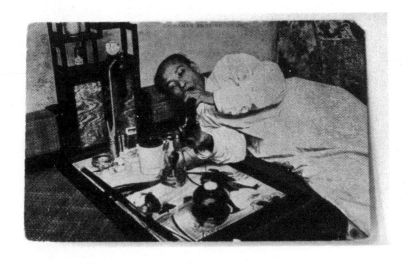

Chinaman Smoking Opium
3½″ × 5″ photo postcard. $20.00

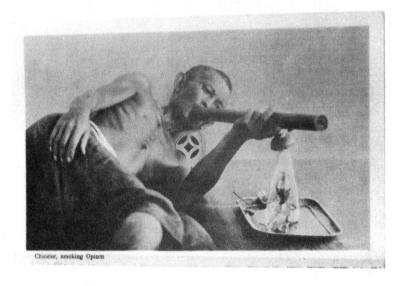

Chinese, Smoking Opium
3½″ × 5″ black and white photo postcard. $25.00

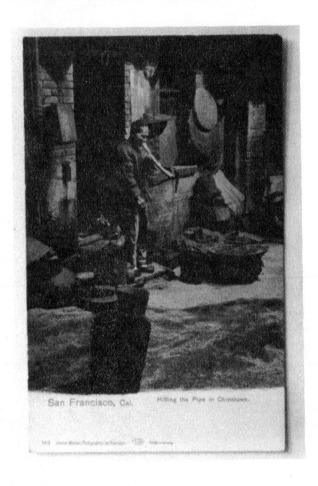

Hitting the Pipe in Chinatown
3½″ × 5″ color photo postcard. Charles Weidner, Photographer.
San Francisco. $20.00

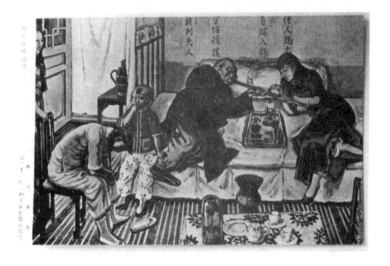

Mother and Father Smoking Opium With Children Present
3½″ × 5″ color painting postcard by artist, Shogo Taguchi.
$20.00

POSTCARDS

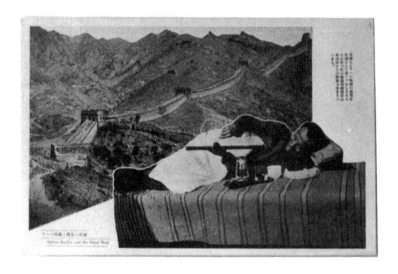

Opium Smoker and the Great Wall
3½" × 5" color photo postcard. $20.00

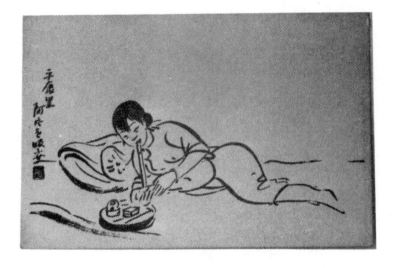

Oriental Female Smoking Opium
3½″ × 5″ artist's sketch postcard. Published by Manchurian
Motor Transportation Co. $20.00

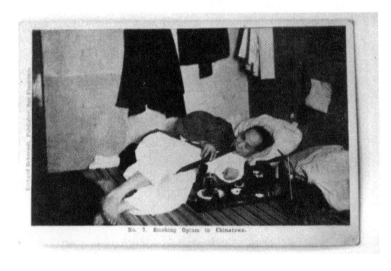

Smoking Opium in Chinatown
3½″ × 5″ color photo postcard. Richard Behrendt, Photographer.
San Francisco. $20.00

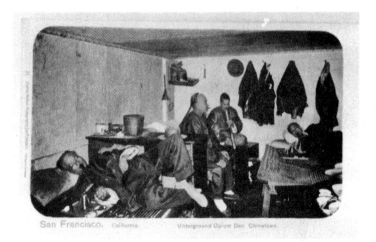

San Francisco. California.   Underground Opium Den Chinatown.

Underground Opium Den Chinatown
Charles Weidner, Photographer. San Francisco. 3½″ × 5″ color
photo postcard. $20.00

POSTCARDS

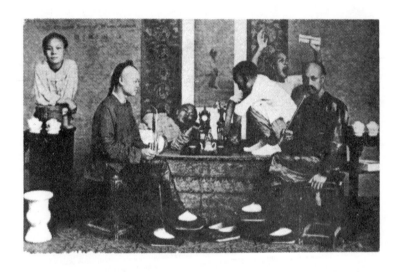

Upper-Class Chinese Smoking Opium
3½″ × 5″ color photo postcard. $25.00

DRUG ANTIQUES CATALOG AND ~§BOOK⁊~

If you would like to receive a catalog of drug antiques and collectibles available for sale, please send $2.00 to:

Cape Ann Antiques
P. O. Box 3502
Peabody, MA 01960

Also if you would like other copies of this book, they are available by sending $12.95 plus $2.00 postage and handling to Cape Ann Antiques at the above address. Dealer inquiries are welcome.

ABOUT THE
❧AUTHOR❧

Jed Power is the owner-operator of Cape Ann Antiques, the first business specializing in drug antiques and collectibles. He publishes a quarterly catalog of drug antiques available for sale. He also welcomes readers' comments and suggestions about this book.